PICTURES IN AIDUCATION

"African Communities Talking Sex, AIDS and Pictures"

Dr Edwin Mavunika Mapara

Order this book online at www.trafford.com/07-2591
or email orders@trafford.com

Most Trafford titles are also available at major online book retailers.

Special thanks for specific pictures used: 1. Picture 1: UNAIDS
2. Picture 6: Richard Tedder, Middlesex Hospital, UK
3. Picture 9: The AIDS Pathogenesis Research Unit at the Burnet Institute, Australia
4. Picture 13: The peer educators in Kenya (Picture 1) and Zimbabwe (Picture 2)
5. Picture 14: Patient from Chinhoyi, Zimbabwe
6. Picture 15: Mike Toole
7. Picture 17: The WHO Safe Injecting Global Network
8. Picture 18: The many African women in the pictures

Note for Librarians: A cataloguing record for this book is available from Library
and Archives Canada at www.collectionscanada.ca/amicus/index-e.html

ISBN: 978-1-4251-5757-9

*We at Trafford believe that it is the responsibility of us all, as both individuals
and corporations, to make choices that are environmentally and socially sound.
You, in turn, are supporting this responsible conduct each time you purchase a
Trafford book, or make use of our publishing services. To find out how you are
helping, please visit www.trafford.com/responsiblepublishing.html*

*Our mission is to efficiently provide the world's finest, most comprehensive
book publishing service, enabling every author to experience success.
To find out how to publish your book, your way, and have it available
worldwide, visit us online at www.trafford.com/10510*

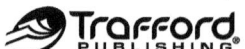

www.trafford.com

North America & international
toll-free: 1 888 232 4444 (USA & Canada)
phone: 250 383 6864 ♦ fax: 250 383 6804
email: info@trafford.com

The United Kingdom & Europe
phone: +44 (0)1865 722 113 ♦ local rate: 0845 230 9601
facsimile: +44 (0)1865 722 868 ♦ email: info.uk@trafford.com

10 9 8 7 6 5 4 3 2 1

Dedicated to the healthcare workers at Athlone Hospital,
The Athlone family, The Athlone Hospital Advisory Committee
and The Community of Lobatse, Botswana.

CONTENTS

Routes of transmission

PREFACE

It has taken quite a while to write down my experiences of working in African hospitals and communities in an HIV infection and AIDS environment. It is not easy as a general doctor or physician based in the government hospitals or health facilities in Africa to write books and papers, for others to read and to learn from as *"gakhuna nako* (there is no time)."

African medical doctors are usually hands on, multi-skilled and one is generally an all rounder in the hospital. This involves performing all specialities and includes being a physician, a surgeon, an obstetrician, a gynaecologist, a paediatrician, a pathologist, a public health specialist, an anaesthetist, an administrator, a health promoter, a teacher and once in a while a politician as one works in the district hospitals.

That reminds me of an instance when I was once an ambulance driver in the hospital, as we ferried burnt bodies from a scene where there had been a terrible fire. We had two drivers on call that night and I became the third driver as Athlone Hospital's Disaster Preparedness Programme was called into action under the guidance of Dr. Jimmy Kununka, the Chief Medical Officer at the time, as he manned the triage and gave commands. Dr Kununka was to Disaster Preparedness as Dr Mapara was to AIDS Awarenes, passionate and focussed. Meanwhile other doctors, nurses, paramedics and general workers were receiving the casualties and treating the fire victims in Athlone Hospital's make-shift Accident & Emergency (A&E) ward. A monthly disaster preparedness drill routine had become a reality. Athlone Hospital excelled on that night.

If this book, PICTURES IN AIDUCATION, will in a world of HIV infection and AIDS

…teach you a fact or two on HIV infection and AIDS as public health disasters,

…inform, educate and empower you to run AIDS awareness projects and programmes,

…help to reduce the stigma and discrimination that is sadly associated with HIV infection and AIDS,

…make HIV infection which is invisible to become visible,

…enlighten people on the history of the Lobatse, Botswana, AIDS Programmes,

…inspire and encourage others to do better than the gold standard set at Athlone Hospital,

…impact on you the value of local African human resources and programmes,

…impress on you the richness of African sayings to relay messages,

…help turn a "brain-drain" into a "brain-gain" as Africa cries for its healthcare workers,

…encourage you to set up a health resource centre in your area,

...instil into others that the use of images or pictures in HIV infection or AIDS education (AIDucation) is a viable teaching method and intervention strategy then it will have served its purpose.

This book is not a scientific or medical textbook. It is simply a true African experience or story on the use of pictures or images in raising HIV infection and AIDS awareness in the community. *"Seeing is very different from being told,"* says an old African saying. There are African lessons to be learnt and African lessons to be unlearnt.

The first part of the book gives a background about the author, a bit of history on two documented district hospitals' *"...best practices...,"* namely Livingstone Hospital Anti-AIDS Project in Zambia and Athlone Hospital AIDS Awareness Project in Botswana. It also gives a bit of background on the "Pictures in AIDucation" teaching style.

The second part of the book is about sharing experiences from Athlone Hospital's AIDucation workshops that primarily discuss Teaching aids At Low Cost (TALC) clinical slides or medical illustrations. This second part would be better understood by reading **"HIV Infection – Virology and Transmission (Africa) HIVT-F Slides 1-24 (November 2002)** prepared by Dr Cathy Vaughan and Wendy Holmes, Centre for International Health, Macfarlane Burnet, Institute for Medical Research and Public Health, Melbourne, Victoria, Australia. The resources are distributed by Teaching aids At Low Cost (TALC), St Albans, United Kingdom. I would have loved to have the coloured pictures in the book, but due to printing costs the twenty four pictures are in black and white. Twelve of the twenty-four pictures have been used in the cover design to give you a flavour of the actual TALC pictures. The English say, *"Seeing is believing!"* The Africans say, *"Seeing is very different from being told!"*

The third part of the book is about Athlone Hospital's *"...best practice..."* Health Resource Centre followed by the fourth and final part, the story of the early days of Botswana's Antiretroviral Therapy Programme and Athlone Hospital's role. Athlone Hospital played a key role in community mobilisation at local and national levels. It is about documenting valuable history lest we forget.

My gratitude goes to all our friends living with and affected by HIV infection and AIDS, AIDucation workshop participants, Athlone Hospital staff and Professor David Morley who have urged me to make a contribution towards this cause by writing down my experiences.

Dr Edwin Mavunika Mapara

ACKNOWLEDGEMENTS

There is a Botswana saying that says, *"Motho ke motho ka batho ba ba ngwe (A person is a person, because of persons around him)."* I am what I am because of the wonderful hospital staff at Athlone Hospital and the community of Lobatse in Botswana. My sincere gratitude goes to the following:

The Athlone Hospital Advisory Committee comprised of Mma Mbulawa, Mma Phuu and the late Patron Mr Goolam Asmal, may his soul rest in peace (MHSRIP) for the *"seed money"* and support that saw Athlone Hospital's AIDS Awareness Project grow from a local *"...alarmist ...noisy...stubborn"* project into a national, respected *"consultancy"* and institution.

The former Hospital Management Team comprised of the Chief Medical Officer Dr Jimmy Kununka, Matron Makhabenyana and the Principal Administrator General Moetedi who gave the Athlone team the freedom to dream local dreams that turned not into one or two but three national *"best practice"* programmes.

The former Honourable Minister of Health in Botswana Mrs Joy Phumaphi, The Deputy Minister of Health Ms Tsiang, The Under Secretary, Mr Ndibi (Ministry of Health), Mr Leonard Manthe (Technical Support Services), Ms Monica Tselayakgosi (National AIDS Coordinating Agency) and Ms Lydia Matebesi (United Nations Development Programme) for the support given to the Athlone Hospital in the later years.

The former Hospital Superintendent of Nyangabgwe Hospital in Francistown, Dr Habaudi Njiro Hobona, for encouraging the Athlone Hospital Team during its early "rough" days, when friends were few and hard to come by.

The former Member of Parliament for Lobatse, Comrade Nehemiah Modubule for the strong, visible political support. Despite being in the leading opposition party, the Botswana National Front (BNF), he whole-heartedly supported Athlone Hospital's AIDS Awareness Programme.

The University Teaching Hospital Medical School lecturers in Zambia for the medical education and training that created the author. First and foremost on the list is Professor Anne Bayley for introducing me to the science of HIV infection and AIDS with a passion. Secondly, I want to thank Professor Chifumbe Chintu and Professor Kopano Mukelebai for encouraging us, as medical students, to believe in ourselves and to treat and look after the community as *"...you would treat your mother, father, brother, sister, children and your extended family."*

Dr Charles Mambwe, Dr Paul Sidandi and staff at the Lobatse Mental Hospital for the support during the teething period of Athlone Anti-AIDS Project. I also thank the Lobatse Mental Hospital healthcare workers for the psychological, emotional and physical support given to the clients and patients living with HIV infection and AIDS.

Dr Vitalis Chipfakacha, the AIDS guru and *"AIDucator"* who coined the word *"AIDucation"* and the phrase *"Get AIDucated!"* All credit goes to him, for the heads that turn or nod at this appropriate terminology. Thank you again for the massive support during our times together.

Dr Diana Dickinson in Gaborone and Dr Kgosi Mompati in Francistown who introduced me to the science of antiretroviral therapy before the Botswana government programme started providing antiretroviral therapy to its citizens. Thank you again for looking after my many clients living with HIV infection and AIDS that were referred to them from Lobatse.

Dr Paul Sidandi, Dr Clement Chela, Dr Christopher Chembe, Mr Onyewuchi Obirieze, Mr Vuyo Mphande, Mrs Anne Esilaba, Mr Bart Esilaba and Mr Isaiah Banda for their loud thoughts and commenting on the manuscript.

The very patient and motherly, Mrs Tuelo Mphele based at Ministry headquarters for teaching me about culturally appropriate health promotion strategies. In the same vein I thank the highly principled *"Coach"* Segolame Ramotlhwa, for his honesty and unparalleled integrity in conducting Ministry of Health business. I thank both of them for their support when I found myself in some trouble, while passionately driving the AIDucation programme. The two colleagues never saw a *"Zambian"*, they saw an AIDucator.

Mmapula Sechele, the former Matron at Princess Marina Hospital in Gaborone for initiating and leading the Athlone Hospital *"National Tour of Hope"* in 1997.

Mr David Ngele and Mr Billy Mosedame (MHSRIP) of Botswana Network of People Living With HIV infection and AIDS (BONEPWA), Reverend Edward Baralemwa of Botswana Christian AIDS Intervention Programme (BOCAIP) and Anne at Total Community Mobilisation (TCM). These team leaders mobilised their teams within two weeks of being called upon, to begin the antiretroviral therapy AIDucation programme rolling-out with the Athlone Hospital Team in Lobatse.

The *"A - Team"* made up of Boile *"Dimples"* Kgaodi, Virginia (Mokopakgosi) Mavura, Phana Mokganedi, Francinah Letlapa, Vaja Ntingana, Proctor Motsime, Maureen Gabalape, Dorothy Keokgale, Nancy Modisaotsile, Yvonne Moatlhodi, Yvonne Matloane, Tsolofelo Afithile, Ronald Molosiwa, *"Phaks"* Mothlake, Alice Mogorosi, Baldwin Khupe, Sam *"Mr President"* Kolane, Andrew Motsamai and William Bapati.

Tirelo, the *"still pictures"* camera-man from the catering department and Joseph, *"the moving pictures"* video camera-man, from the supplies department for documenting and recording Athlone Hospital's AIDS Awareness Project history and life.

Others who made our *"AIDucation Away Days"* successful were Molly Keoreme and Maggie Matsake, from the industrial class, who handled the catering very well and made delicious homely meals. I miss the seswaa, serobe and the salads. Those local community hall AIDucation sessions were always successful social intercourses that broke barriers between the staff. Those sessions had no doctors, nurses, paramedics or industrial class. They had the "Athlone family."

The "portables" in the typing-pool, namely Nunu and Matau for their patience in typing the loads of AIDucation materials.

The men at Athlone Hospital for the "...men to men..." talks as we discussed intimate sexual matters. The men, mostly in the Transport office, are Rre Sharp Knowledge, Rre Motoroko, Rre Mokgano, Moses, Martin, Michael, Counsellor Shimane, Richard, Thabo and Rre Selepe.

Kenneth, the driver from Princess Marina Hospital must not be forgotten for driving the Athlone Team, from Lobatse to Maun and safely back to Lobatse during the 1997 first national assignment, *"National Tour of Hope."*

His Excellency President Festus Mogae and His Excellency the Vice President, Ian Khama for giving me the opportunity to work on the "Original ARV Team" that laid the foundation for the Botswana Antiretroviral Therapy Project. That call up was a challenge that I have cherished to this day, as I tell *"The Botswana ART Story"* at my annual lectures at the London School of Hygiene & Tropical Medicine, University of London.

Mrs Noerine Kaleeba the Founder and Director of The AIDS Support Organisation (TASO) of Uganda for encouraging the team to "...*continue your good works. It is just a matter of time."* She rightly predicted, during her visit to Botswana in June 1995 that Athlone Hospital would become a national programme *"...that others will learn from."*

Dr Cathy Vaughan and Dr Wendy Holmes for the permission to reproduce the AIDucation manuals, especially the twenty-four pictures. This book would not have been possible without these resources, as this book is literally *"a feedback on the TALC slides"* at the request of Professor David Morley. "*Zikomo kwambili (Thank you very much)"* Dr Vaughan and Dr Holmes whole-heartedly, for the permission to use the Teaching aids At Low Cost materials.

Glen Williams and Alison Williams of Strategies for Hope Trust, Oxford, for their support and for the Oxford couple introducing me to the world of HIV infection and AIDS in London.

Professor David Morley for my first publication, *"Picturing AIDS: Using Images to Raise Community Awareness"* and for literally reminding me, every other day, to put pen to paper for *"...this exciting abuse of the TALC slides..."* and for the *"...fantastic stories that these slides have generated."*

Emily Bell for the memorable invitation to the World Health Organisation (WHO) headquarters, Geneva, in December 2004, for an AIDucation experience with the AIDS experts. I thank Emily Bell again for one of my greatest historical moments in my life, of taking part in Nelson Mandela's birthday party celebrations at Hyde Park on 27th June 2008. Agatha (my wife) and I were part of the 46 664 invited guests. *"Yebo!"* Thank you!

Anne Francis in Norwich, for her motivation and infectious positive outlook to life and for supporting AIDucation.

Teaching aids At Low Cost (TALC) staff, St Albans, for their fantastic work that involves distribution of these resources to the developing countries. Some of the tribes in Africa who have watched and discussed these pictures would say *"Asante sana! Taonga! Twalumba! Twatasha! Merci! Gracias! Danke! Keitumetsi! Webale nyo! Yebo! Zikomo! Thank you!"*

The Community Health Action Trust (CHAT) team and the many wonderful volunteers led by the Director, Mr William Gemegah that gave Pictures in AIDucation a chance.

Reverend Jefferson Kwamina Crystal for remembering us in his daily prayers, and for reminding us daily that, *"The Lord is good"* in his morning greetings.

My mother- Mrs Gertrude Mapara and my mother - in-law, Mrs Sabina Mulenga who gave us the permission to, *"follow your dreams"* as we said good-bye to Africa.

Posthumously, I thank my father, Mr Frackson Robert Mapara and my father –in-law, Mr Paul Mulenga, for the *"seeds"* they planted and nurtured. May the souls of the two departed men rest in eternal peace.

Finally, but not least my special gratitude goes to my wife Agatha Mapara and the boys - Masuzyo Robert Mapara, Temwani Christopher Mapara and Claude Mukuka Mapara who many a weekend were left on their own as I went on AIDucation missions in Africa and now in Europe.

To the many others, I have met on this long journey and did not mention by name, I say *"Yebo!"* Thank you!

The views, comments and facts in this book are not representative of any African government, hospital or voluntary organisation. I take full responsibility for all the written work with the main aim of "AIDucating" communities in HIV infection prevention, care and support activities.

There is a Zambian saying that says, *"When you run alone, you run fast. When you run together, you run far."* I trust that we shall run together and learn together as I tell my story. Another wise African saying, says, *"When you have learnt, you must teach."*

Dr Edwin Mavunika Mapara

PART 1

African sayings in Pictures in AIDucation

- *"Motho ke motho ka batho ba ba ngwe."*

(A person is a person because of persons around him).

- *Seeing is very different from being told.*

- *The ruin of a nation begins in its homes.*

- *Before one cooks, one must have the meat.*

- *You must judge a man by the work of his hands.*

- *Knowledge is like a garden, if it is not cultivated it cannot be harvested.*

- *Death is like a robe that everyone has to wear one day.*

- *Great events may stem from words of no importance.*

- *One who enters the forest does not listen to the breaking of the twigs*

- *Smoke does not affect honey-bees alone, honey gatherers are also affected*

- *A picture is worth a thousand words.*

- *Until the lion has his own story teller, the hunter will always have the best part of the story being told.*

- *It takes a village to raise a child.*

- *You have to look after wealth, but knowledge looks after you.*

- *It is the calm and silent water that drowns a man.*

- *When you run alone, you run fast. When you run together, you run far!*

African writers

1. INTRODUCTION

> *"The ruin of a nation begins in the homes of its people."*

African saying

The impact of HIV infection and AIDS

The world was relatively *"at peace"* in terms of public health disasters or diseases, although preventable infections such as diarrhoea, malaria and tuberculosis kill millions of people each year, in the developing countries. The "peace" was and is no more with the entry of human immunodeficiency virus (HIV) infection and acquired immune deficiency syndrome (AIDS) that have brought a lot of suffering, misery, devastation, poverty and death in many homes, especially in sub-Saharan Africa. As from the early 1980s, a lot of dreams in terms of family life, growth and development have been shattered by the arrival of HIV infection and AIDS, the two public health disasters of untold proportions and magnitude.

Very few, if any, African families in sub-Saharan Africa have not had a death in the family or attended a funeral of a relative, friend, neighbour, work colleague, church or mosque congregation member who has died of AIDS. Death has become a *"normal"* daily event, with thousands of Africans being buried every single day across the continent. Death has *"become acceptable"* in many families as we bury the dead and wait to bury the dying. Death has dried up the tears of many people who have cried their tears dry, as life seems to have no meaning any more. Death still remains a mystery, difficult to comprehend and difficult to understand to the mere mortal.

Grandparents that have lived their lives are being called upon by AIDS to re-live their young days again by not only nursing their sons and daughters, but by also taking over the responsibilities of bringing up the orphans and the grand-children as the parents die. Weekends that used to be for weddings, celebrations, joyful social outings and parties are now mostly for conducting funerals, burials and comforting the bereaved.

AIDS has taken away the bread-winners, disrupted families, destroyed education, damaged industries, dislocated health services, ground agriculture and threatened world security. AIDS is every where in the communities.

The rich, brown, sweet smelling African soil is swallowing up its sons and daughters before the prime of their lives, as they sleep their last eternal sleep. In some communities there are even debates of whether to bury or to cremate, as burial sites and the many graves take over potential arable, farmlands and future commercial plots. Burial sites are now strategically placed on the outskirts of towns or villages for the expected fast expansion as more people are still to die expected natural deaths and predicted unnatural, avoidable deaths.

Statistics or numbers do not mean much to a lot of us. To understand the gravity of the situation in Africa it is best to relate the HIV infection and AIDS epidemics to the Twin Towers' disaster or the Tsunami disaster. How many people died in those two very unfortunate tragedies? It is *"...not African to talk of the dead"* but in this case our fore-fathers will have to forgive us as we try to picture a point to the world about what HIV infection and AIDS has done to the African continent. In the developing countries, between the cock crowing to call up the yellow sun to rise and the evening golden sunset, we are witnessing three *"Twin Towers' disasters"* every single day, that is close to 9 000 deaths per day or 63 000 deaths per week or 252 000 deaths every month.

How many "Tsunami" disasters (deaths) occur in Africa in a year? There is almost one in every month and therefore twelve "Tsunamis" per year.

Impact on health services

With HIV infection and AIDS we are forced to *"...think the unthinkable, say the unsayable, sometimes predict the unpredictable, imagine the unimaginable, visualise the invisible, picture the unpicturable and do the undoable or manage the impossible,"* according to one AIDucation workshop participant. With the amount of death and suffering that we were seeing in the hospitals, in Zambia and Botswana, business could not be conducted in the usual manner. We had to do something to ease the suffering of the patients, first and foremost. Secondly, counselling services had to be put in place for the healthcare workers who were being mentally affected or burnt out. The hospitals were teaching about HIV infection and AIDS prevention in the community and already caring for the sick and the *"waiting to die"* AIDS patients as there was no treatment or cure.

The profession of Medicine was no longer an exciting profession. That joy of seeing patients heal, rise and walk out of hospital was slowly being replaced by sadness, frustrations, hopelessness and the feeling of failure. Healthcare workers felt the agonising pain when discharging bedridden patients on stretchers, to go home for home-based care and to literally wait for death, *"...as the hospital has done its best and the rest is now in God's hands."* That is what it was bluntly. It was even more painful to *"create"* bed-spaces for patients with curable diseases and *"discharge"* those with incurable diseases. Were healthcare workers displaying double standards? Were we being hypocrites? Were we discriminating? Were we increasing the stigma that we were striving to reduce? Some angry relatives to the discharged patients felt that *"...doctors and nurses are playing Modimo (God)...deciding who dies and who lives."* Healthcare workers had become cruel.

AIDS was in the village. We were beginning to bury in bigger numbers, although many people would not openly talk of the cause of death. Living with HIV infection or AIDS had its stigma and it was believed that the client or person infected with HIV infection or living with AIDS *"...has brought shame"* to the family. Families were judgemental. It was all about *"...loose morals...running around...having many sexual partners... promiscuity ...immorality ...infidelity"* and all the *"wrong"* sexual behaviours. One could die of anything else, but not HIV infection or AIDS in those early days. Many patients died lonely deaths because of the shame, stigmatisation, depression and isolation.

Some clients or people living with terminal AIDS would even request the healthcare workers to *"...please end my life... end my suffering... put me to rest in my final sleep...relieve me from this torture!"* These requests came mostly from patients with severe cancers that were slowly *"...eating up"* their bodies. The most common cancers were of the anal region, the women's private parts and Kaposi's sarcoma, a cancer of the blood that affects the whole body. Others had terrible bedsores or pressure sores or big wounds, which were as a result of the patient not being nursed or looked after properly.

Bedridden patients have to be moved or turned over frequently so as to allow free blood circulation to all the parts of the body, during home-based care. Athlone Hospital always advised the care-givers to routinely turn over the patients every two hours or moved about to exercise the limbs and increase the blood circulation. This was an easy instruction, but difficult to carry out by many relatives or care-givers for various reasons.

To many seriously ill patients the pain and suffering was unbearable and life was not worth living. As some clients said dejectedly, *"...it was hell on earth!"* Before the arrival of antiretroviral therapy relatives had no alternatives but to silently watch and pray as patients died, and in some cases, such terrible, painful, agonising and embarrassing deaths.

Families painfully watched their loved ones wither, shrivel or shrink to the extent of where they were literally *"...skin on bones...human skeletons...finished."* Parents watched their sons and daughters age over weeks or months to become *"...old people"* as the youthfulness vanished and HIV infection turned energetic bodies into full-blown tired, weak AIDS' bodies. Parents looked physically younger than their daughters and sons, while the sons and daughters being nursed looked like the parents to the parents. How do you explain such a situation to the grand children, who at times looked on with fear? Many children witnessed the lives of their parents drain away as they questioned Him above, about his unconditional love, tender mercies and mysterious ways of *"...God gives and God takes"* and *"...God takes all the good people!"*

There is no euthanasia or *"mercy killing"* in Zambia and Botswana. All that we, the healthcare workers, could do was to reduce the pain and suffering and make the patients' hospital stay as comfortable as possible (palliative care). Similarly we would also do the same for home based care clients, to make their last days on earth, at home, with the family as comfortable as possible.

Slowly and surely many a hospital in Africa has *"shifted"* into the homes with the relatives learning how to be healthcare workers. Hospital drips (intravenous fluids) were being set up in the homes. Not an option but a necessity in Africa and other developing countries, as many healthcare workers left and leave the continent for *"greener pastures"* or simply changed professions so as to *"...have a break from the suffering"* being witnessed in the homes and hospitals. To some of the healthcare workers it was and is a way of coping and managing "burn-out" as the smell of death lingered on in the air, reminding all and every single day of HIV infection and AIDS. One of the most difficult procedures was to shut the eye-lids, prepare and take the body of a fallen colleague to the mortuary and await burial. Healthcare workers are not immune to HIV infection or AIDS and they are affected like everyone else. HIV infection and AIDS are not selective, we are all at risk.

Africa does not have the luxury of too many care-givers or carers, nurses and medical doctors. It is not *"...breaking news"* to hear of one doctor looking after a population of 20,000 or 100,000 people. In Lobatse, Botswana, we had on average five government doctors to a population of 32,000 people and meaning that almost one doctor to 6,400 people. Botswana is one of the better off countries in terms of human resources or health personnel and can better embrace the concept of *"Health for All"* by the year 2016.

In some rural areas in Africa, the health facilities are run by hard working nurses or recalled, retired nurses. In some other remote areas health facilities are becoming *"white elephants"* as the number of healthcare workers dwindle and the centres are left alone to ponder what once was.

It was reported by World Health Organisation (WHO) in 2006, that Africa needs about 1 million healthcare workers to address the current health problems on the continent. At the same time it was reported that 20,000 healthcare workers leave Africa for the West every year. With these disturbing facts, Africa has no choice but to train all the community members that it can in basic nursing care so that they can nurse their own patients in their homes. This used to happen in the past and it has to happen in the present times. Cruel as it might sound, it is reality, dictated by HIV infection and AIDS, the brain-drain and critical shortage of resources.

The lack of healthcare workers is one of the many reasons used for justifying the teaching of village folks through Pictures in AIDucation. Athlone Hospital was simply preparing the community for what was still to come - diseases not seen before, unbearable suffering, hospitals in the homes, change of roles and responsibilities between parents and children, torment, misery, new HIV infections in the hundreds and deaths due to AIDS in the thousands.

This book, firstly, is about living in a real world where HIV infections and AIDS related diseases dictate the way of life, both in the rural, traditional villages and in the urban, modern cities and towns. This is a real story for the Livingstone and Lobatse families for their faith, trust and confidence in what we did as a town or village team. As the saying goes, *"Motho ke motho ka batho ba ba ngwe (A person is a person because of persons or people around him)."*

The author owes the success of "Pictures in AIDucation", which we shall simply call or refer to as *AIDucation,* to the people of Livingstone and Lobatse, who had the faith in the *"small doctor"* and *"mosimane (boy) doctor"* respectively. Where words or sentences in the story are written in *italics,* means the words are direct quotations from the many community members that the author related with or had a social intercourse with in the last twenty-five years in a world of HIV infections and AIDS in Zambia, Botswana, South Africa, England and Switzerland.

This story is a *"feedback"* in response to Prof David Morley, who asked for a *"...feedback on how you used the slides (TALC) in Africa..."* at my first public AIDucation presentation in London.

Meeting with Professor David Morley

I recall the first day I met Professor David Morley in January 2003, at the Institute of Child Health Seminar: **"Role of Print and Visual Media in the Management of HIV infection and AIDS in sub- Saharan Africa."** It was a wonderful and a memorable day for me. It was officially the continuation of Pictures in HIV infections and AIDS education (AIDucation), the London chapter.

On coming to London in August 2002, for my postgraduate studies in Infectious Diseases, I had promised to keep my mouth shut on HIV infections and AIDS related matters and focus on my studies. I did not want to be distracted from my school work, especially that age was not on my side and this grey and white matter needed tender loving and care (TLC), to compete with the young brains in class.

I had been involved in HIV infections and AIDS programmes in Zambia since 1985 and then in Botswana, from September 1990 to August 2002. The plan was to keep quiet until after obtaining my Masters degree in 2005. I did manage to keep quiet, but only for three months. Along came Glen Williams, the editor of Strategies For Hope (SFH) Series, in October 2002 and the rest is history.

After almost twenty years of involvement, teaching with pictures in AIDucation, I truly believe that we have *"missed the boat"* in teaching and reaching communities on matters involving sexual health and sexually transmitted infections, including HIV infections and AIDS. We have not *"pictured"* sexual and reproductive health. This has been my belief for the last twenty-five years and I came to a definite conclusion after my first seminar in London, at the Institute of Child Health, where I met Professor David Morley.

In my first public audience in the United Kingdom, there was one Head of a Health Promotion Department, from a prominent London Medical School who commented after the Pictures in AIDucation presentation. She was fascinated with the use of colour images in AIDucation and she asked, *"Have we misled the public? Have we misled ourselves? Do we need to revise the Health Promotion curriculum?"* There were no answers to these simple and difficult questions, but a loud silence as all thought deep and hard as they looked at this African from Zambia and Botswana who was on the stage humbly challenging the status quo.

I had gladly shared my experiences of working in Zambia and Botswana with the university lecturers and students. My aim as I spoke was to turn a *"...brain-drain"* into a *"...brain-gain"* which was very possible. This has partially happened as I am frequently invited to *AIDucate* volunteers, consultants and various non governmental organisation' members, who go to Africa to give a helping hand in caring for and supporting people living with HIV infection and AIDS.

While on stage, during my presentation, I was amazed at seeing this elderly man literally beaming in the front row of the audience as he listened to my talk. I could not understand the happiness and visibly excited expression of this gentleman. I noticed only one face in that sea of white faces and few black faces at the Institute of Child Health - this beaming, physically visible, very happy person. I became a bit confused and wondered at what was so exciting that I was saying to cause this individual in the front row to be so elated. After the presentation I sat down. The old man was looking at me, smiling with satisfaction and very impressed at something. I was baffled.

I quickly scribbled a note to Glen who was seated next to me on the stage as we faced the audience, *"Glen, who is this old man wearing spectacles seated almost opposite me in the front row?"* Glen scribbled back the reply, *"How do you use somebody's slides and you do not know him?"* It was my turn to display unexplained emotions and was stunned at the possibility of who this person could be. I recalled the authors' names of the Teaching aids At Low Cost slides or AIDucation pictures that I had used in Botswana since 1992. The AIDucation pictures were made by Dr Cathy Vaughan, Dr Wendy Holmes and Professor David Morley. The first two authors were ladies, from the names and this was a man in front of me. I scribbled my surprise back to Glen, *"Professor Morley!?"* Glen wrote back, *"YES. Professor David Morley!"*

I could not believe the coincidence. My first public lecture, my first AIDucation audience in London, England was in front of the owner of the TALC slides, *"Athlone pictures,"* as the

AIDucation pictures were popularly known as in Botswana. This was *"The"* David Morley of *"Morley's Textbook of Paediatrics"* and *"My Name is Today,"* that I was looking at from the advantage point of the stage of the Institute of Child Health. I was looking at the President and Founder of Teaching aids At Low Cost, the organisation which he had created in 1965, in his house, in England. I was five years old by then, in Zambia, preparing to start my education in Grade one at Lusaka Infants School. Here was the man whose *"TALC movement"* was reaching almost every corner of the earth, especially in Africa, with the subsidised health educational materials. Here was the man who had made the hospital I came from, Athlone Hospital in Lobatse, Botswana, the *"international"* HIV infections and AIDS programme that it was at that time. To think that since 1983 it was only the name I knew as a medical student in Zambia. Now there I was in January 2003, almost twenty years later having visibly impressed Professor David Morley, the child (Paediatrics) guru himself. What a coincidence for AIDucation and a pleasant surprise.

When Professor Morley came over to congratulate me for the *"... fantastic ten years feedback on the old 1989 TALC slides..."* I was dumbfounded and bewildered. While still recovering from the surprise, he invited me over to St Albans, the home of TALC to *"...pick up the 2002 edition of the slides."* I quickly accepted the invitation, without the slightest clue on earth of where St Albans was or how I would get there. That was secondary and not an issue at that moment. The important issue was the gospel truth that there I was having a dialogue with the internationally renowned Paediatrics Consultant, Professor David Morley in person.

I usually tell friends who are not in the field of Medicine that sitting with Glen Williams and Professor David Morley was almost the equivalent of sitting next to two famous footballers like Pele of Brazil and Beckham of England in the world of football.

My teaching life or health promotion has been with colour pictures, so naturally I sent my colleagues in Africa the four pictures that I took at St Albans with Professor David Morley. That did the trick. *"Seeing is very different from being told."* The pictures were taken on the day I went over to meet the powerful TALC Team and also to have my time tested 1989 TALC slides replaced by the modern 2002 new slides.

The TALC Team has and continues to work wonders for many individuals, couples, families, tribes, schools, churches, companies, institutions of higher learning and grassroots community based organisations in Africa. Gratitude goes to the TALC team for the six sets of TALC slides that were given to me, when I visited St Albans. The slide sets were sent to fellow healthcare workers in Zambia and Botswana. One set of pictures went to Livingstone General Hospital, Zambia, where my AIDucation sessions began and five sets of pictures went to Botswana, where the AIDucation sessions matured. The recipients in Botswana were The Family Health Division, Gaborone; Ministry of Health, Gaborone; Kanye Seventh Day Adventist (SDA) Hospital; Bamalete Lutheran Hospital, Ramotswa and naturally Athlone Hospital, Lobatse.

I hope that my story will inform, AIDucate and help to empower many people on HIV infection and AIDS matters in both the developed and the developing countries.

The author, Dr Edwin Mavunika Mapara, on the left, pictured with Professor David Morley at TALC headquarters, St Albans, London, United Kingdom.

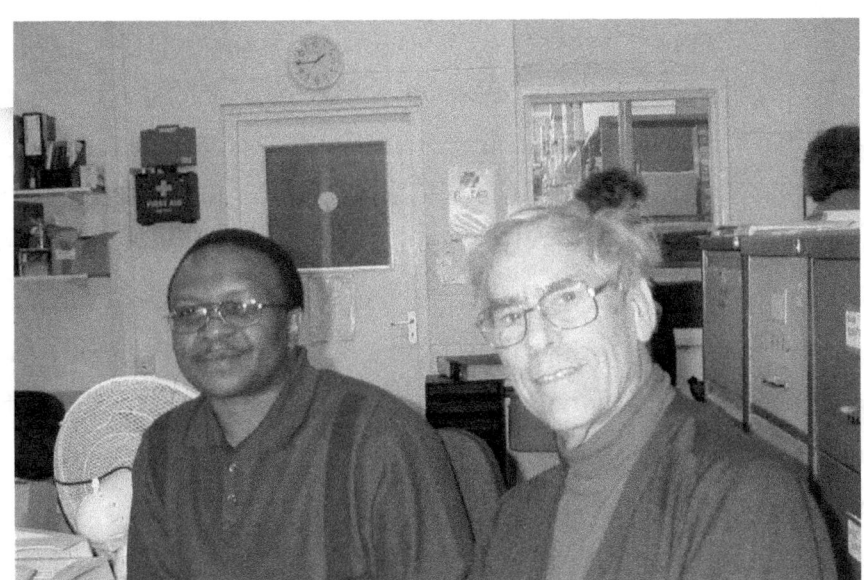

DR EDWIN MAVUNIKA MAPARA   28

Feedback on the use of TALC pictures

Professor Morley had asked for a feedback on how I had used the TALC slides or *"AIDucation pictures"* that were made by his team that included Dr Wendy Holmes and Dr Cathy Vaughan. We are talking of close to twenty years of showing hospital or clinical images in AIDucation to grassroots organisations. The AIDucation pictures have been used in close to two-hundred workshops, seminars, lectures and conferences in Africa and Europe. Where does one start from to answer the *"...feedback on TALC pictures"* question? As they say, *"Start from the beginning."*

I will start with an introduction of myself. It is not easy to introduce or talk about oneself, so I will use the words that the Chairman used to introduce me in January 2003, the month I gave my first public talk at the Institute of Child Health, where I first met Professor David Morley. After the introduction I will then give some relevant, sexual related background information from Zambia, Botswana and other African countries that will make understanding the feedback much easier.

About the author

"Dr Edwin Mavunika Mapara was born on the Copperbelt town of Kitwe, in Zambia, where he spent his early years. The family later moved to Lusaka, the capital city of Zambia. His primary, secondary and university education were all in Lusaka. He studied Medicine at the University of Zambia (UNZA), where he graduated with a Bachelor of Science in Human Biology (BSc.Hb), and a Bachelor of Medicine and Surgery (MBChB). He later obtained a Diploma in Tropical Medicine and Hygiene (DTM&H) at Witwatersrand University, South Africa, in 1998.

In 2002, Dr Mapara re-located to the United Kingdom where he is currently studying for a Master of Science in Infectious Diseases at the London School of Hygiene and Tropical Medicine (LSHTM).

As a medical student, in 1985, Dr Mapara helped to look after one of the *"first"* early officially diagnosed and recorded AIDS patients admitted at the University Teaching Hospital (UTH) in Lusaka, Zambia. The patients were admitted under the surgical firm of Professor Anne Bayley, a renowned authority on Kaposi's sarcoma and who was Dr Mapara's mentor and lecturer. Professor Anne Bayley of Yellow Firm, Surgery Department, had noticed something *"...unusual..."* in 1983 about the patients presenting with Kaposi's sarcoma, a cancer of the blood. That was just the beginning of the sad story that would affect every Zambian family in one way or another.

The year 1985 was the land-mark "initiation" year for Dr Mapara into HIV infection and AIDS initiatives, projects and programmes that would span more than two decades. He worked on the Yellow Firm, University Teaching Hospital, under the firm, uncompromising Professor Anne Bayley. He says that one had no choice but to know in depth all the facts on Kaposi's sarcoma, HIV infection and AIDS, while on the Yellow Firm.

Since then Dr Mapara has been credited with the formation of, *"...best practice(s)"* in Zambia and Botswana - the Livingstone Anti-AIDS Project, Zambia 1989; The Athlone Anti-AIDS Project, Botswana, in 1990 and the Athlone Health Resource Centre, Botswana, 1999. The health resource centre is being replicated nation wide by the Botswana government and its many international partners. This is evidence of what Dr Mapara believes is an example of a *"good practice"* African programme being born, developed and implemented in a small district hospital, where there were no consultants, but just local general doctors, with a passion to make a healthy difference in the local community of Lobatse.

Dr Mapara has facilitated and presented in several workshops, seminars and conferences in Zambia, Botswana and South Africa. He has received several Public Health awards and accolades.

21

Dr Mapara advocates for the use of colour images or pictures in HIV infection and AIDS education, which he has dubbed *"Pictures in AIDucation"* to raise awareness as *"Seeing is very different from being told!"* He believes that colour images or colour pictures stimulate dialogue, initiate debate, provoke emotions, address denial, simplify complicated facts, show reality, create rapport and clarify information where medical jargon has failed. He believes that pictures make it easier to introduce discussions on culturally sensitive *"...taboo..."* subjects of sexual intercourse, sexual relationships, sexuality and death. *"Pictures in AIDucation"* breaks the silence and makes people talk. The ultimate fact is that AIDucation facilitates empowerment. As the Zambian saying says, *"A person with a mouth cannot get lost!"* It is all about using the mouth and the eyes. It is all about asking, talking, dialogue and discussions aided by colour pictures.

Dr Mapara, on graduation from University of Zambia (UNZA) Medical School in 1987, worked at the University Teaching Hospital (UTH) in Lusaka, Zambia. He then moved on for his district posting in Livingstone, Zambia, where he worked until September 1990. As fate or destiny would have it, Dr Mapara had registered for his postgraduate studies at the London School of Hygiene and Tropical Medicine (LSHTM) and was supposed to start classes on 24th September 1990, to study for his Masters in Tropical Medicine. Unfortunately at the eleventh hour the scholarship was withdrawn and that was *"...the beginning of the end of Dr Mapara in Zambia and the beginning in Botswana of Dr Mapara."*

Heart-broken and disappointed at the prospect of not coming to this *"great school"* for his postgraduate studies, Dr Mapara left Zambia for Botswana, where he worked for a good twelve years. He says that going to Botswana was a blessing in disguise. Today, he comes to London School of Hygiene and Tropical Medicine with a vast experience, from the African continent, of active involvement in HIV infection and AIDS control programmes.

Dr Mapara worked diligently in Botswana on the HIV infection and AIDS control programmes, laying the foundation for Athlone Hospital's future international status in HIV infection and AIDS management.

Dr Mapara was appointed the Chief Medical Officer of the 175 bed district hospital, Athlone Hospital based in southern Botswana, in the Lobatse district, in 1997. He was a *"consultant"* in HIV infection and AIDS matters for the Botswana government and many non-governmental organisations. In 2001, he was appointed to head the Clinical (Medical) unit of the newly formed Antiretroviral Therapy Programme that would provide treatment or therapy to the citizens of Botswana who were living with HIV infection and AIDS.

After contributing to the birth of the first largest African government sponsored antiretroviral therapy programme and the roll-out to the four selected sites of Gaborone, Serowe, Francistown and Maun, he left Botswana in August 2002 for London to pursue further academic studies, challenges and to market Pictures in AIDucation.

On that note I will call upon Dr Edwin Mapara to share his experiences as a Medical doctor who has been in the front-line of the sub-Saharan HIV infection and AIDS epidemics."

The introduction was a bit lengthy, but maybe it was justified as I was a stranger in town, coming from Lobatse, Botswana, about ten thousand miles away on the African continent, which many people would not have heard of or read about.

With that introduction, there is very little more to say about myself. The only update is to state that I am through with my postgraduate studies, Master of Science (MSc) in Infectious Diseases and have graduated.

I have been involved in various aspects of HIV infection and AIDS prevention, care and support activities for close to twenty-five years and I have worked in both, the hospital and community set-ups, consulting, teaching and sharing experiences on HIV infection and AIDS with pictures. I have been very successful in raising awareness amongst the grassroots communities by using or rather *"abusing"* the Teaching aids At Low Cost clinical pictures. I am not blowing my trumpet, but simply stating or rather picturing a fact.

Teaching with colour pictures

The visual resources used are of sexually transmitted infections, HIV infections and AIDS clinical manifestations. These were made for training or AIDucating healthcare workers - medical students, health educators, nurses, paramedics and doctors.

It is a fact that there is no better teaching method to use than colour pictures or images when talking to ordinary people in the village about sexually transmitted infections. The visual impact lingers on for years, as compared to written materials that disappear or are forgotten after a few months. That is why Athlone Hospital went one step further than Teaching aids At Low Cost to use or rather abuse the AIDucation pictures to AIDucate the non-health, non-hospital and non-science community members in the village. The pictures worked wonders with the African communities in raising awareness on sexually transmitted infections. After all we already have been told that, *"...a picture is worth a thousand words"* and Athlone Hospital was only putting that old English saying into practice. With twenty years of picturing HIV infection and AIDS, take it from me, that it is true that, *"...a picture is worth a thousand words"* and that *"...seeing is very different from being told."*

23

Past target audiences

Picture the following groups of people viewing and discussing the AIDucation pictures; Teachers in their schools, civil servants in the offices, soldiers in the barracks, the police at the police station, pupils and students in primary and secondary schools, college and university students, church congregations with their ministers, pregnant mothers at the ante-natal clinics (ANC), traditional birth attendants and traditional doctors in the community halls. The list is endless of community members who have viewed and discussed these pictures.

As time went on and more community members became knowledgeable and empowered through pictures in AIDucation, there was a backlash. Quite a number of the folks were not impressed with Athlone Hospital, for not having used the AIDucation pictures to raise awareness, *"...when government started talking about AIDS in the early 1980s in the village."* The question *"Why?"* was frequently asked by the African participants, after the AIDucation sessions.

This same question was and is also being asked in London, after Pictures in AIDucation sessions at Brent by the European participants. I am sure that the American, Asian, Australian and Russian AIDucation participants would ask the same question, *"Why aren't the other AIDucators teaching with pictures?"*

AIDUCATION

AIDS stands for Acquired Immune Deficiency Syndrome. Note that AIDS and Human Immunodeficiency Virus (HIV) infection are two different conditions. You can have HIV infection but not have AIDS.

Blood transfusion of unscreened blood or blood products may spread HIV infection.

2. COMMUNICATION AND CULTURE

"Before one cooks, one must have the meat."

African saying

Talking about sex

Teaching or talking about sexually transmitted infections including HIV infection and AIDS can be quite a challenge in the developing countries. There are some medical terms that are just not there in the vernacular or local languages. Interpretation of languages also dilutes some meanings of messages in some cases, or gives ambiguous meanings and even nonsensical meanings.

To add to the difficulties of communication, HIV infection and AIDS is about sexual intercourse, sex education, sexuality and death, which in most developing countries are culturally sensitive *"no go areas"* or *"taboo"* subjects. This has resulted in people not being informed, AIDucated or empowered early enough to learn and understand the basic life saving skills and scientific facts on HIV infection and AIDS, that can bring about behaviour change. Many people are still being infected today out of ignorance, despite the wealth and volumes of information available. This *"...new disease"* is still *"...very invisible"* in many villages and towns.

Furthermore, *"...Good Africans...Africans with good manners...civilised Africans...Africans brought up in proper, decent homes...people with a culture...God fearing people..."* are brought up not to talk about sex. This (im)moral teaching, in a world of very serious sexually transmitted infections, is right across the African continent and it has cost the African continent precious human lives and time. Africa has paid dearly for its silence on AIDS with thousands of highly skilled, semi-skilled and casual labourers being buried or cremated daily, as AIDS silently reaps the silent African communities.

"Silence is golden"

There are instances or situations where *"silence is golden"* but not with HIV infection and AIDS. Silence has cost the African continent and other developing countries. Silence has fuelled the spread of HIV infection and AIDS. Silence has led to procrastination, stigma, discrimination and isolation. We have to talk, talk and talk about sex, no matter how embarrassing it may be. We have to picture, picture and picture sexually transmitted infections, if we are to survive as a human race. We have to break the silence if mankind has to avoid extinction. Many homes, villages and towns have been left empty, in what the westerners term *"ghost towns"* because the occupants have all died or moved away as a result of HIV infection and AIDS.

I passionately believe that empowerment with Pictures in AIDucation usually leads to change in attitudes and risky behaviours. Written information alone, and there is plenty of it going around, does not seem to make much of a difference. Is it time to picture HIV infection and AIDS? Is it time to picture tuberculosis (TB)? Is it time to picture the ill health of smoking? Is it time to communicate public health messages through colour pictures? Pictures lead to dialogue. Pictures lead to health promotion. Pictures lead to empowerment. Pictures lead to health, safety and security. Pictures do not portray the same messages as words. Pictures are more powerful as AIDucation resources.

The AIDucation teacher

The messenger, teacher, facilitator or carrier of the AIDucation messages into the community makes a huge difference. Empowerment is best facilitated or led by local community leaders who know the language, culture and way of life of the local people. The local village chiefs, headmen, elders and leaders are respected gatekeepers of African traditional values, culture and sexual matters. They are the *"doors"* into those thousands of homes, bedrooms, villages and towns. We must work with the traditional leaders if we are to successfully AIDucate the many culturally diverse communities in the developing countries.

The faith community leaders are key *"movers and shakers"* in African communities on issues of moral discipline and decent behaviour. These leaders are important in one to one, or face to face contact with community members. Africans are *"deeply spiritual"* and that is a point that we have missed when discussing HIV infection and AIDS. We, as healthcare workers, were very slow to bring the faith communities on board and have contributed to the Bible passage that states that, *"My people die due to lack of knowledge."*

African culture and spirituality plays a major role in effective AIDucation communication in Africa. Humans are sexual beings. Humans are spiritual beings. Have we used these two facts in our communities when talking about HIV infection and AIDS? Communication is about knowing the sexual culture of a people. Communication is about knowing the spiritual beliefs of a people.

"Oral history" is still an effective communication tool in addressing HIV infection and AIDS. People silently cry *"Talk to us!"* We, Africans, are still a continent of *"...observations, oral history and story-telling!"* Sadly, the traditional community leaders, gatekeepers and church leaders, who are looked upon by their subordinates, have not been utilised to the fullest in curbing the spread of HIV infection. They have been marginalised or brought into the fold too late. Who is better than the owner

of the house to know its occupants, practices and activities happening in the bedrooms? Who is better placed than the faith leaders or pastors to know their faith communities and flock?

Information dissemination and leadership

What has happened in many African communities has been wide information dissemination by the many local healthcare workers and foreign consultants, with little consultation or involvement of the local people or natives of the land who are affected. The results have been obvious, a public health disaster of untold magnitude, as the locals do not own these programmes.

Like many other nationals, Africans too are a proud lot despite their documented poverty, turmoil, upheavals and many undocumented African born successes and programmes such as Livingstone AIDS Awareness Project (Zambia); Athlone AIDS Awareness Programme (Botswana), Pictures in AIDucation (Botswana), Athlone Hospital Health Resource Centre (Botswana) and Community Resource Centre (England). Africans have survived where many would have succumbed. Africans generally do not like people doing things for them, just like many non-African communities, especially where it involves changing our cultural ways of life. We prefer to work together or slightly have the upper hand, the edge, which is human nature in one's home, bedroom, village or country.

What does the Chinese saying say about how a fish rots? *"A fish starts rotting from the head!"* Using this in the African HIV infection and AIDS situation, I believe that most public health programmes that have failed have had poor leadership that lacked vision. Those programmes that tried to stop the spread have had a very strong political leadership. Look at the "good" results of Uganda, Zambia and now Botswana, where HIV infection and AIDS is being controlled, mainstreamed and new infections reduced or prevented. Despite the denial and delay in response to address the epidemics in the initial days, the political commitment has been second to none in these three African countries led by President Yoweri Museveni (Uganda), President Kenneth Kaunda (Zambia) and President Festus Mogae (Botswana). These three noble men took the bull by its horns, as the English saying goes. These honourable men have done Africa proud.

Another great name, AIDS activist, to be added to the list is Nelson Mandela of South Africa. I was there at Hyde Park on 27th June 2008, to see this great African hero celebrate his 90th birthday with Gracia, his wife, by his side. My wife Agatha and I were part of the 46 664 ticket holders at Hyde Park that evening, with compliments of Ms Emily Bell who I met through AIDucation in London. Nelson Mandela, despite his 27 years behind bars, has done a lot in terms of AIDucation, care and support for people living with HIV infection and AIDS in South Africa.

27

"It is in your hands," was the AIDS message by the great Nelson Mandela on the night of 27th June 2008. Stop reading this book for a minute and look at your hands. What have you done to address the AIDS situation in Africa? What can you tell Nelson Mandela about your role and activities in containing the spread of AIDS or supporting people living with HIV infection or living with AIDS in your country? *"It is in your hands,"* says Nelson Mandela. It was a fantastic birthday celebration with all those other great celebrities and musicians.

Cultural practices that fuel spread of infections

There are some traditional rituals or practices that have helped fuel the spread of HIV infection, AIDS and other sexually transmitted infections in Africa. Some of the practices include:

1. **The culture of silence**

   Sexual intercourse, sexuality, the penis, the vagina and the anus are not talked about. These are *"taboo"* subjects or *"unspeakable"* words. Not discussed, period.

2. **Wife inheritance or spouse inheritance**

   When the sexual partner or husband has died, the widow or spouse has to be *"inherited"* by a family member who has been *"...delegated the responsibility of looking after the woman, her children and family property."* Part of the process involves *"cleansing"* and this is performed sexually with no condoms used. It is believed that the sexual act *"...releases the spirit of the dead sexual partner or spouse."*

   Sadly, I know of cases where the women insisted that they be *"set free"* through this ritual, despite having the full knowledge that their husbands or partners died of full blown AIDS. This is criminal for lack of a better word. The English people would arrest the person with HIV infection in London, *"...for knowingly or deliberately spreading the virus"* and be charged with *"...Grievous Bodily Harm (GBH)"* which carries a ten years jail sentence.

3. **Sexual intercourse with a young virgin**

   There is a strong belief that a man who is HIV infected can have his *"...HIV infected blood cleaned or purified by having sexual intercourse with a young virgin."* It is believed that the younger the girl, the better the cleansing or purification process. This is not true.

   This barbaric belief is sadly still being practiced or taking place in some countries. The scientific fact and gospel truth is that when one has HIV infection it is for life. HIV infection cannot be cleaned, drained, sucked or washed out of the human body. It dies with the body.

4. Polygamy

This is the culture where a man has many wives. It is still quite a common practice in some communities. I know of families where there was trouble when HIV infection was brought into the families sexually. I was called upon and involved in trying to settle some *"disputes"* that arose due to this polygamous arrangement. Naturally other sexual partners within the circle became infected through marriage and sharing the husband or the man.

5. Traditional circumcisions

When young men become of age in many African communities they are taken to traditional initiation camps where they are circumcised and welcomed into manhood. The *"blade"* used for cutting the fore-skin of the penis of the initiates is anything from a sharp stone, piece of glass bottle, razor blade, knife or spear. The instruments used might be shared amongst the young men and might be poorly cleaned. Lack of sterility of the circumcision blades is a major issue in these traditional camps.

I am for male circumcisions. I support male circumcisions but very opposed to the traditional, none sterile way of doing or performing them. Many communities do it for cultural or religious reasons. Circumcisions are best done in hospitals or clinics under clean, sterile conditions. Arrangements for hospital circumcisions are not difficult when the health authorities are approached.

Male circumcisions reduce chances of acquiring sexually transmitted infections by 60%, as we were taught at medical school in the 1980s. This fact remains true today.

6. Female genital mutilation (FGM) or female circumcision or female genital cutting

This is a very controversial subject. This traditional practice is more common in North and West Africa than Southern Africa. Female circumcisions are done on social grounds, religious grounds or on hygienic grounds. The wound created can lead to infections, including sexually transmitted infections. It can also be a source of many future complications when the time comes for sexual intercourse and child birth.

7. "Blood letting" by traditional doctors

Some people believe that *"...bad blood...sick blood...HIV infected blood"* can be removed or drained from the blood system. *"Blood-letting"* is done by some traditional doctors. Some traditional doctors use their mouths to suck the *"...bad blood"* from the clients, after cutting or making some incisions, *"elevens"*, into the clients' arms, legs or other parts of the body.

Some traditional doctors use the horn of a cow or tennis ball to *"...suck the bad HIV blood."* Some traditional doctors cut through patients' haemorrhoids or piles and let them bleed to get rid of the *"...bad HIV blood"* in the client with HIV infection or AIDS. A number of these patients have ended up with complications and had to be admitted to the local hospitals, for doctors to attend to. I know of some traditional doctors who have died with HIV infection or full blown AIDS. Did they contract HIV infection through sexual intercourse or was it through these traditional *"bloody"* procedures that they acquired HIV infection or AIDS?

The "cultural approach" and the "spiritual approach" in AIDucation

It is important to have a *"cultural approach"* and a *"spiritual approach"* to addressing HIV infection and AIDS in Africa. Take note that quite a number of these "outlawed cultural practices" are slowly dying away in Africa, as people become more and more educated, enlightened and AIDucated. Many young people or the new generations do not even know of some of these practices and therefore do not practice them or promote them.

There are some good African traditional practices that we should keep and pass on to the young generation. The outlawed African traditional practices that can cause us harm must be done away with, especially those that involve sexual intercourse, those that involve the penis and the vagina. Traditional leaders must look into these dangerous intimate practices.

The author has deliberately left out the very intimate African sexual practices that he learnt about in the many AIDucation workshops held over the years. The intimate sexual practices learnt about are from Botswana, Kenya, Malawi, Namibia, Rwanda, South Africa, Swaziland, Tanzania, Uganda, Zambia and Zimbabwe. These sexual practices will be discussed at a later date as we open up and freely talk about sex and sexuality. Meanwhile ask around while waiting for the next book, AIDucation in Pictures.

We have to seriously talk about HIV transmission and the main route of transmission in Africa, which is through sexual intercourse, mostly through the penis inserted in the vagina.

African sayings and HIV transmission or spread

Different people have different ways of expressing themselves or relaying messages to others. Africa's niche or strength in relaying messages or teaching valuable lessons is found in rich, old African sayings. The elders have a way of teaching lessons using these proverbs or sayings. The majority of sayings are good, with hidden valuable meanings or messages.

A few of the African sayings have to be re-visited. There are some sayings or proverbs that tend to promote the transmission of sexually transmitted infections, including HIV infection. These sayings are said or talked about in a certain way that give the picture or impression that it is alright for a man to have more than one sexual partner. Some of these sayings are:

- *"On the hand, it is only the thumb (man) that can touch the other fingers (women)"*
- *"For an axe (man) to become sharp, it must chop down many trees (women)"*
- *"For a bee (man) to make honey, the bee must touch pollen from many flowers (women)"*
- *"When your husband comes home late, you must not ask him questions about where he has been"* is common advice given to the new bride at wedding ceremonies.

To prevent new HIV infections we must address the bad and unhealthy practice of having several or multiple sexual partners or *"...links"* as I have been taught by the youth of Brent in London. A person having sexual intercourse with multiple partners or *"...links"* helps in the spread of HIV infection and other sexually transmitted infections. Similarly he or she is also prone to catching other sexually transmitted infections from the same multiple sexual partners or "links" in the community.

African names and their meanings

Still talking on the subject of culture and away from HIV transmission, let us talk about names. Yes, the meanings of African names. Many traditional African names have a meaning and can be an entry point into talking about sex. As the English say, *"One man's meat is another man's poison!"*

The author's name has a unique meaning, depending on which side of the Zambia-Botswana border one resides or lives on. The Christian name is Edwin, followed by the middle name given at birth, Mavunika and Mapara is the family surname. When literally translated in the author's mother tongue, which is Tumbuka, the name Mavunika means a *"breech presentation"* or born with legs first. Usually babies are born with the head (cephalic presentation) first. The name Mapara means *"many bald heads"* or many human heads with no hair on them.

Crossing the southern border of Zambia into Botswana, the meaning is completely different. In Botswana, Mavunika means *"to break"* or *"to cover"* and Mapara means *"area (perineum) between the legs where we have the penis or the vagina!"* The author tells folks that, that is why he talks freely about sex, the penis and the vagina. He is licensed or rather named to talk about the area between the legs and the contents or *"goods"* or *"parcels"* in the area. Some elderly folks in Botswana failed to say or mention the name *"Dr Mapara"* as it was *"...an insult... vulgar... obscenity...too heavy for the tongue..."* and therefore preferred to call him *"Dr Mavunika."* As if that was not enough in a name, a Dutch medical doctor at Athlone Hospital once asked the author, *"How come all your names are sexual?"*

31

Coming to London, the author had one of the Batswana ladies fail to explain his (Mapara) name to her English colleague in one of the big churches, where the author was a guest speaker as the congregation prayed for Southern Africa and its public health problems, especially HIV infections and AIDS, in June 2005. The Motswana sister said to her friend, *"I cannot tell you the meaning of his name (Mapara) in Church. I will tell you outside!"* The author's name could not be mentioned in the House of the Lord. That is what deep embedded respect, spirituality and culture can do to the African woman and man. The English pastor had no problem mentioning Dr Mapara more than six times in the church service. It was just a name of a person. I wonder how the church would have responded had he said it in the Setswana interpretation or version, *"Dr In between the legs!"*

I usually use *"Mapara"* to break the ice or create a rapport during AIDucation workshops. I would usually, during AIDucation workshops, pick out some other *"interesting"* names to *"break the ice"* or to get people talking about the *"sensitive and embarrassing"* subjects of sexual intercourse, sexuality, the penis, the vagina and the anus.

The next time you run a workshop in the African communities ask for the meanings of those African names. You will be surprised at what you will learn. Africans are named after events, happenings, family members, relatives, week days, important historical dates or body parts, like in my name. Another thing about some African names is that the same family, under the same roof or house-hold may have different surnames, yet the children all have the same biological father and the same biological mother. Why? That is how it is culturally.

Here are some African names met in the AIDucation workshops with their meanings;
Bupe (Gift), Chimwemwe (Happiness), Kalala (One who sleeps), Kanyama (Small animal), Lorato (Love), Natasha (I am grateful), Naledi (Shining star), Modisaotsile (The shepherd has come), Moeng (Visitor) and Motsumi (Hunter).

There are only two million African names left for you to interpret. Good luck!

AIDUCATION

Cure has not been found for HIV infection or AIDS to date. However there are some anti-HIV drugs or antiretroviral therapy that improves the quality of life of people living with HIV infection or AIDS. These drugs are taken daily and are for life. No drug holidays.

Diagnosis of HIV is by a reliable HIV blood test. Challenge yourself and get tested. It takes a man to be tested. It takes a woman to be tested. You have more to lose by not knowing your HIV status. Make the right choice. The HIV test is in your hands. Take the test! Why wait?

3. COMMUNITY *"BEST PRACTICE"* PROJECTS

"You must judge a man by the work of his hands."

African saying

District posting at Livingstone General Hospital, Zambia

I left the University Teaching Hospital (UTH) in Lusaka in August 1989 after completing my internship and that was two months after my wedding in June 1989. I served my one year district posting and had my wedding honeymoon in Zambia's leading tourist town of Livingstone, the home of one of the most magnificent water falls in the world, the Victoria Falls.

The other day on British Broadcasting Corporation (BBC) television I saw *"The World's Strongest Man"* competition being held in Livingstone, Zambia. It brought back sweet and sad memories of my home-town; the sweet memories, in terms of its happy, smiling people, the beautiful weather, the priceless natural organic foods and sadness in terms of the hardships and difficulties that AIDS had brought.

I was based in Livingstone, from August 1989 to September 1990, where I helped to form the Livingstone Anti-AIDS Project. The original project team was made up of ten members. These included hospital staff, two members from The Zambia Red Cross and a Catholic Sister or nun. Livingstone Anti-AIDS Project was made up of ingredients from the internationally renowned Chikankata Salvation Army Hospital AIDS Programme, in Zambia and The AIDS Support Organisation (TASO) of Uganda, set up by Dr Ian Campbell and Mrs Noerine Kaleeba respectively.

The Livingstone Project was composed of the units of Information, Education and Communication (IEC), Counselling, Clinical Care, Home based care, Pastoral Care, Integrated Training; Research and Administration Units. This modified model would later on be used in Botswana.

The Livingstone Project used the popular early 1980's Uganda HIV infection and AIDS posters to teach on HIV infection and AIDS. The posters made a big difference in sharing information with the communities, but we were still not communicating effectively. We were struggling to get some messages across about this *"...invisible illness..."* that affected *"...bazungu (white people)..."* The Livingstone Anti-AIDS Project added drama and song to the community intervention strategies to raise HIV awareness and to engage people into dialogue and looking after their health. *"Beat the drums and the people will come"* was advice given by the drama group. The drums were beaten. The people came. We engaged them after sketches and songs on HIV infection and AIDS.

The Livingstone community response to the public health messages was positive with the formation of school anti-AIDS clubs and the formation of AIDS at the workplace programmes. Initially the Livingstone workplaces, especially the factories and industries were reluctant to invite the Livingstone Anti-AIDS Project team. The team told the managers of the workplaces of what HIV infection and AIDS was going to do, not might do, to their work forces in the years to come if action was not taken straight away. The picture painted was very grim, honest, pessimistic and convincing.

The factories and companies accepted the team, but *"...only in the afternoons..."*, so that the team did not, according to the workplace administrators *"...disturb our morning operations...we run on profits...we have no time to waste on talks!"* The team did not respond to such comments, as time would tell, naturally. Time did tell and productivity in many companies started going down as HIV infection and AIDS struck down workers, disturbing the workplace operations, productions, the profits and the growth of the companies.

The district of Livingstone began talking HIV infection and AIDS in the schools, workplaces, churches, market places and community gatherings. The Livingstone Project got the politicians talking on HIV infection and AIDS in all their public talks and engagements. This was made easier for the project team by the strong political support from the District Governor, at that time, who was a military man. He told all the politicians in Livingstone to put in *"...at least 10 to 15 minutes talk on AIDS..."* in the speeches they were delivering. He was firm and rarely smiled. When he gave an instruction or rather military order, very few, if any, would not obey.

Livingstone newspapers in AIDS activities

Everybody has a role to play in addressing HIV infections and AIDS. The local media in Livingstone played a major role in community sensitisation and mobilisation. The media was a strong partner to the Livingstone Anti-AIDS Project. The Livingstone Anti - AIDS Project team was frequently making sensational headlines in the national newspapers, with the Livingstone community HIV infection and AIDS activities.

The *"best"* newspaper story was written by one of the local journalists of a national paper, The Times of Zambia. He wrote an article on one suggestion that one of the Livingstone Project team members had made, during a brain-storming session on how to raise awareness in the surrounding villages. The suggestion came as a question. *"Why not distribute an information package in the villages that has HIV infection and AIDS leaflets for AIDS control, Oral Rehydration Salts (ORS) leaflets for diarrhoea treatment and High Energy Protein Supplements (HEPS) leaflets for treatment of malnutrition (kwashiorkor) with the census teams that will be moving from door to door?"* This brilliant suggestion was made by a young hospital X-ray attendant who had never seen the four walls of the inside of a secondary school classroom.

It was a brilliant idea, but it came too late. Can you imagine the national response had we done that at a national scale in 1990, in all the nine provinces of Zambia? We did not know at that time that the Americans had carried out such a similar door to door campaign in the early 1980s, although it ended up a national disaster. It was later found that the Americans watched more television than read health information leaflets or pamphlets. *"Seeing is believing"* and *"...seeing is very different from being told!"* Maybe the Americans should have used Pictures in AIDucation at that time on television.

In early 1990 the Livingstone AIDS Awareness Project received a telephone call from the Permanent Secretary of Ministry of Health on the *"...noble suggestion of health information spread through the Census programme."* He telephoned Livingstone Hospital after he read an article in the national newspaper, describing Livingstone Hospital's initiatives. The call came in the morning, at a time when I was conducting a TB ward round in Batoka Hospital, Livingstone.

One of the nurses came running into the ward with the urgent message from the Permanent Secretary, Ministry of Health headquarters. I went to answer the call wondering what crimes I had committed, for headquarters to call me. Whatever it was, I had a feeling it was to do with the AIDS programme as some policy-makers did not like my *"...alarmist and frightening"* style of raising community awareness on AIDS. I was very right.

I received a telling off or was castigated for not having suggested *"...the brilliant information distribution strategy earlier on for all the nine provinces to do!"* The Livingstone Anti-AIDS Project story was on the front page of one of the newspapers, again. Initially I did not know what the Permanent Secretary was talking about, as Livingstone, which was almost 420 miles away from Lusaka, received the daily morning newspapers in the afternoons with the first buses from Lusaka that set off at about 6.00am. Livingstone heard of the fantastic story in the morning but saw the *"Census story"* in the afternoon.

We thanked the Livingstone journalist for his positive contribution that got the Livingstone community talking and more interested to engage with the Livingstone Project in addressing HIV infection and AIDS. The media can break or make a programme. The Livingstone Anti-AIDS Project was fortunate that the media were its friends in Livingstone, Zambia. This was going to be the same, later with the Lobatse media in Botswana where destiny had already planned my future. Responsible, mature positive media reporting is a plus for all the people who are trying to help to make a positive contribution to bringing HIV infection and AIDS under control.

I thank all the editors, reporters and journalists that I have worked with, in Africa, for their positive AIDucation input. They built the Livingstone and Lobatse district AIDucation programmes. They played the role of *"The Good Samaritan on the road from Jerusalem to Jericho"* in a world of people living with and affected by HIV infection and AIDS.

AIDS control projects in district hospitals

Some of the best health promotion initiatives come from the rural areas, villages or district hospitals. This was so with Livingstone Anti-AIDS Project in Zambia and later on Athlone Anti-AIDS Project in Botswana. Why is this so? District hospitals usually do not have the luxury of urban hospitals and learn to adapt and make do with what they have in terms of limited resources. This is a *"blessing in disguise"* in its own ways. The local community is one of the strengths or unique resources of district hospitals when it comes to public health and community mobilisation. That is how, both, the Livingstone Project, in Zambia and the Athlone Project, in Botswana utilised the multi-sectoral approach to raise HIV infection and AIDS awareness in the communities. We needed more people to be involved. We simply called them and they happily came.

Multi-sectoral simply means working with the many sectors in the community. Multi-sectoral means working with everyone. These sectors include the civil service, trade unions, faith communities, schools, media, politicians and other non-governmental organisations to engage the people in HIV infection and AIDS prevention, care and support programmes. The AIDS awareness projects in the districts were already talking *"multi-sectoral approach"* and *"mainstreaming AIDS"* because of the limited resources. There is an old African saying that says that, *"One hand cannot clap. It takes two hands to clap."*

By 1990, the Livingstone Anti-AIDS Project was being discussed in the same vein as the Copperbelt Health Education Programme (CHEP) and the Lusaka based Schools' Anti-AIDS Programme. The Livingstone media put the Livingstone team in the lime-light and won the team respect and followers for the innovative ideas. If the media could write more stories on local public health programmes, it would help all of us to look after each other's health.

The *"...downside"* of the Livingstone AIDS awareness programme media headlines, according to some politicians was the *"...negative publicity for tourism"* that was spreading in Livingstone, the home of Zambia's tourism industry with the magnificent Victoria Falls, the major tourist attraction. Some politicians thought that the tourism industry would go down and there would be loss of money or revenue from tourism as *"...tourists stopped coming to visit Livingstone and stopped investing in Zambia...for the fear of catching AIDS!"*

The media can be a positive force for change, with proper sensitisation and AIDucation. Lack of AIDucation can lead to careless, insensitive, sensational reporting and like careless talk can be very dangerous. People living with HIV infection and AIDS can simply go under ground and keep quiet, which is the last thing we want to happen. The media in London is the very opposite of the media in Africa, when it comes to reporting on HIV infection and AIDS stories. The negative headlines I have seen and read about HIV infection and AIDS, in London, leave me usually disturbed. I will keep the examples for the next book, *"African Communities Talking Sex, AIDS and Pictures in London"* that will follow shortly.

We have to work together, as the infected or affected, in a world of HIV infection and AIDS. No one is immune to HIV infection or AIDS. Any one of us, including journalists, editors, teachers, lawyers, accountants, pastors, soldiers, pilots, politicians, celebrities, footballers, musicians, traditional doctors, social workers, nurses and medical doctors can acquire or become infected with HIV infection. We are human and we are all at risk.

District posting at Athlone Hospital, Botswana

The author left Zambia for Botswana in September 1990. Recall that the author was supposed to have left Zambia for his postgraduate studies at the London School of Hygiene and Tropical Medicine (LSHTM), University of London, England, in September 1990.

My first and last appointment was at Athlone Hospital in Lobatse district, situated in Southern Botswana, where I worked for the next twelve years, until August 2002. History began to repeat itself in public health. I helped to set up the Athlone Anti-AIDS Project, which we later re-named Athlone AIDS Awareness Project so as to accommodate and embrace all community members, those living with HIV infection and those affected by HIV infection and AIDS. It was simply the Livingstone Anti-AIDS Project re-locating to Lobatse in Botswana.

The Athlone Hospital Project in Botswana was similar to the Livingstone Hospital Project in Zambia. They both suckled from the same breast and both were involved in HIV infection and AIDS prevention, care and support activities. The Athlone Hospital Project was formed in 1990, before the Botswana National AIDS/STD Programme which was formed in 1992. This early birth at Athlone Hospital had its advantages and disadvantages.

Athlone Hospital like Livingstone Hospital AIDS Awareness Project was made up of seven units:

- Information, education and communication (IEC)
- Counselling
- Clinical Care

- Home Based Care (HBC)
- Pastoral Care
- Research and Administration
- Integrated Training Unit.

We called these units *"The House of Hope."* The *"house"* was built on a **strong foundation** of information, education and communication. **The concrete slab** was the counselling unit. The **four walls** of the house were made up of the four units of clinical care, home-based care, pastoral care and the research & administrative unit. **The roof** of the house was the integrated training unit, made up of the individual team leaders of the other units (Foundation, slab and walls). I hope you can visualise or picture the house. AIDucation is about building a house of hope.

Unfortunately some of these units were not there at national level and hence the lack of understanding and support by the Ministry of Health in the early days, when Athlone Hospital was reported to have made some *"...too ambitious demands"* according to the authorities. This negative response, another blessing in disguise, made Athlone Hospital look for all sorts of ways (multi-sectoral approach) to engage the local communities, as the Livingstone Programme had done with the Livingstone community in Zambia. *"Deja vu!"* History was repeating itself.

In Botswana, Athlone Hospital had a leading edge in addressing HIV infection and AIDS matters, with the added *"Zambian touch."* I used to tell the Athlone Hospital team members in the early 1990s that, *"You are seeing HIV infection and AIDS through the Zambian eyes, but you are yet to see your own (Botswana) local epidemic, through your own eyes."* HIV infections and AIDS were silently devouring the unsuspecting communities in Botswana. The epidemics were *"...invisible"* to the eyes of many local people.

By 1994 HIV infections and AIDS were becoming visible and the socio-economic impacts of the two epidemics were being felt. There was evidence in terms of ill-health that *"...something was just not right and not right in a very big way"* as observed by one of my first early clients living with HIV infection. She lived bravely with HIV infection for close to fifteen years. She died before I left Botswana. May her soul rest in ever lasting peace. She died before Botswana began providing anti-HIV drugs in 2001. Many times I look back and wonder how many people would have been alive had African governments boldly started providing antiretroviral therapy much earlier on. There is no need to cry over spilt milk. Life must continue. We are all responsible for what has happened to the African continent by our actions or inactions.

Noerine Kaleeba visits Athlone Hospital

Athlone Hospital's AIDS Awareness Project was made up of ingredients from the renowned Chikankata Salvation Army Hospital AIDS Programme and Livingstone Anti-AIDS Project in Zambia, which AIDS activists, visiting from Zambia noticed when they came to Botswana.

Similarly, visitors from Uganda observed The AIDS Support Organisation (TASO) components in Athlone Hospital's AIDS Awareness Project when they visited Botswana.

The TASO Founder and Director, Mrs (Dr) Noerine Kaleeba, commented on the similarities of Athlone Hospital with TASO when she visited Botswana in June 1995. She was very inspirational to the Athlone team and motivated the team's fighting spirit. She gave the team a group counselling session that was therapeutic and second to none. She was after all the *"mother"* of counselling, not only in Uganda, but in Africa.

She told the team about her life in the early days of HIV infection and AIDS in Uganda, in 1986. She talked about how her late husband was diagnosed with AIDS in England and how he was looked after like a brother and *"...given the love and support by his white friends"* from Terrence Higgins Trust. This is what inspired and motivated Noerine Kaleeba to start her own support group of fifteen people. Today, her support group, TASO, is an international organisation with more than 5,000 branches in Uganda, East Africa.

After almost three hours with Noerine at Athlone Hospital, she encouraged the team to, *"...Keep on with your work. One day your programme will become a national programme. I can see a combination of TASO and the Zambian programme in your (Botswana) programme."* She had been through it and she knew that Athlone Hospital was on the right track. It was just a matter of time, sadly after many new preventable HIV infections and deaths, that Botswana would realise *"...the important role of this small but big Lobatse programme."* True to Noerine Kaleeba's words, in 1997 Athlone Hospital AIDS Awareness Project had become a national programme.

AIDUCATION

Education, AIDucation and more AIDucation is a key intervention strategy in containing the spread of HIV infection. Remember that, *"Prevention is better than cure!"*

Females are more vulnerable to acquiring HIV infection than men due to biological, social, gender, cultural and economic reasons. Women and girls must be protected from abuse. Females must respect males and men must respect women.

4. TEACHING ABOUT HIV INFECTION AND AIDS IN AFRICA

"Knowledge is like a garden, if it is not cultivated it cannot be harvested."

African saying

The North develops AIDS programmes for the South

I have never ceased to be amazed and amused at how HIV infection and AIDS programmes are born or hatched in the developed countries to be implemented in cities, towns and villages of the third world or developing world, where the way of life of Africans is completely different from the way of life of the Americans or English people. Unfortunately many of our leaders were short-sighted and encouraged this behaviour and trend to the detriment of many wonderful, local, home-brewed, culturally appropriate HIV infection and AIDS control programmes.

With the severe social and economic impact of HIV infection and AIDS in Africa, one would expect some very good initiatives to come, naturally, from Africa or the countries affected. Good examples are Zambia's Livingstone Anti-AIDS Project and Botswana's Athlone AIDS Awareness Project, local initiatives that became national programmes, out of persistent stubbornness.

Had I been *"...you must be law-abiding"* and heeded the call by my colleagues *"...to keep quiet...remember that you are a contract officer..."* I do not believe we would have been talking about Zambia's Livingstone Anti-AIDS Project, Botswana's Athlone AIDS Awareness Programme, Botswana's Athlone Health Resource Centre and England's Community Resource Centre based at Community Health Action Trust in the borough of Brent, London. These are all documented *"...best practice..."* programmes in Zambia, Botswana and England.

The projects in Zambia and Botswana were carried out the African way. We knew what had to be done and refused to be swayed by *"foreign"* consultants. The Livingstone and Lobatse public health programmes believed in the local indigenous *"native"* consultants who were infected and affected by HIV infection and AIDS. They lived with HIV infection and AIDS every single day. Their brains and way of life were challenged every single day. The suggestions by the locals, inside the country on how to run AIDS awareness programmes, were more valuable than the suggestions from the consultants outside the country. Sadly, many years later, the *"expensive foreign"* consultants were now being taught by the *"cheap native"* consultants and replicating the natives' initiatives that developed and matured out of stubbornness. What wasted valuable years. What missed life saving opportunities. *"No Need To Blame"* is a Zimbabwean video tape worth watching.

Africa has to believe in its own sons and daughters if it has to grow into an internationally respected *"...AIDS awareness power-house"* especially in the field of health. Some of the best teachers in AIDucation, HIV infection and AIDS Medicine were born, schooled and worked in Africa. Paradoxically, many successful HIV infection and AIDS programmes in America and Europe are run by the same Africans, who are never listened to in Africa, who constitute part of the *"brain-drain"* that is forever blamed for Africa's ills. Can you honestly blame them, hands on heart?

Africa's dependency on foreign consultants

I have always been very amazed and curious about Africa's dependency on foreign consultants. The other day I attended a meeting at Canary Wharf, London, organised by The Young Fabians, where talks were being given by prominent international speakers on what the United Kingdom had given to Africa in terms of foreign aid and donor support. True, the United Kingdom has done quite a lot for Africa in academic terms.

In the same vein United Kingdom has also been very unfair to Africa, with the help of the African leadership in messing up some of the HIV infection and AIDS control programmes. It was interesting, painful, heart-breaking and a shock to hear a response to one of my three questions at the meeting that, *"...Last year, in 2005, the HIV infection and AIDS Consultants from Europe to Africa were paid £220 million!"* The silence that followed the answer in the conference room was deafening. You could hear a pin drop despite the hundred or so participants in the room. I had asked the question about the consultants and their pay deliberately, having entertained all those consultants that came to Africa to teach us, or rather learn from us, on managing HIV infection and AIDS. In fact in that same meeting, there was one young consultant who commented on my question. He addressed me as *"Dr Mapara"* which surprised me as I had introduced myself as *"Edwin"* before asking my three short burning questions from the African soil.

During the drinks and net-working I approached this young gentleman to find out where he had heard or met me before as I could not place his name or face at all. He greeted me in Setswana, the national language of Botswana. That was a clue, but I still could not place him. He then told me of the Consultancy Team that he was part of that came to Botswana in 2002 to do some work for the Botswana Antiretroviral Therapy Project. I still could not picture him in Botswana, until he said, *"You came from a hospital (Athlone) in Lobatse with your pictures to teach us on AIDS!"* Eureka! That rang a bell. I could see him now vividly, as he sat attentively in my class at Family Health Division, Gaborone, Botswana, as I taught the Consultants *"The Basic Facts of HIV infection and AIDS"* using the same Teaching aids At Low Cost pictures that will be discussed in the second part of this book.

Strangely, some of the consultants did not know that there was a difference between HIV infection and AIDS. Not surprisingly, some of the consultants had never heard of the internationally renowned HIV infection and AIDS programmes run by Chikankata Salvation Army Hospital in Zambia, The AIDS Support Organisation (TASO) of Uganda or Terrence Higgins Trust (THT) in the United Kingdom.

Just as there were bad consultants coming to advise the Africans, we had some very genuine, good consultants. We must give credit where it is due as there were a handful of very good consultants who came in from renowned hospitals in America and England who taught us a thing or two from the American and English HIV infection and AIDS Programmes. I believe that the majority of consultants, that I met, learnt from the indigenous Africans. I have lost count of how many times I had to teach or "update" consultants on the African HIV infection and AIDS situations.

A few were humble enough to acknowledge this fact and informed the government(s) of the resources *"...discovered in the district hospitals."* One does not know whether to cry or to laugh when you are described as a *"discovery"* by some young foreign medical doctor or social worker brought in by your employers to show you how to run a serious, life and death, HIV infection and AIDS control project in your district, a topic he barely understands.

I had some foreign consultant friends who were brought in and who would uncomfortably ask after a few days of discovering their level (lack) of knowledge, *"Edwin, who is supposed to be teaching who?"* I would comfortably respond, *"You are supposed to be teaching me! You are the consultant. I am a simple district medical officer."*

Traditional charge or *'penalty'* for lack of respect

Teaching or talking to ordinary people about any health related subject, can be a daunting task or challenge, especially in the developing countries. This is not made any easier by talking about *"sensitive"* topics such as sexual intercourse, sexuality and sexually transmitted infections, including HIV infection and AIDS. Many Africans are socialised not to talk about such *"...intimate issues ...private matters...bedroom issues..."* or *"...adult things."* These are *"...not public matters"* as many an African adult or elderly would say. Words such as penis, testicles, vagina, clitoris, sexual intercourse and homosexual do not come out of the mouth of a *"...well brought up... good mannered... decent and cultured African"* and are unheard of in the public arena.

I got into quite a bit of trouble in the early days in Botswana for allowing my *"...bad mouth"* to talk on these matters or utter the forbidden words. I was reported to be *"...insulting"* the village elders by not only talking about these genital organs, but also showing pictures of these *"...private parts"* as part of Athlone Hospital's AIDucation discussions. I was guilty and charged quite a few chickens for *"misbehaving!"* That is a traditional way of reprimanding people who break tradition or transgress. More serious crimes can even be punished by the elders requesting for a bull or a cow to be paid to them. That is a very hefty fine and definitely leaves an empty pocket when the fine is paid.

Similarly many Africans do not talk about death or dying. It is a taboo subject. It is an omen. Cultures do not allow it unless you want to *"...insult the elders..."* who are the gatekeepers of culture and traditions or you want to *"...disturb the ancestral spirits."* People do not even mention the names of the deceased, lest *"...you disturb their sleep!"* You talk of *"...the departed...the late"* or *"...the deceased."* No names mentioned. In the West it does not seem so. The dead are always brought up and discussed as if they were still alive. The late *"...people's princess"* (MHSRIP) in England has never rested, by African standards. It is also customary to say *"May her or his soul rest in peace"* after referring to the dead.

I was once told by a respectable village elder in the early 1990s to *"...keep away from these matters of sex and death!"* That was after Athlone Hospital had conducted AIDucation workshops on *"Good Dying and Good Death"* at the local community hall. There was an outcry in the village, as folks could not understand what was *"good"* about death and dying. I was called a witch or is it a wizard? *"What type of a person talks about good dying and good death, apart from a witch?"* There are times when *"silence is golden"* and this was one of those times... for a few minutes, I must add, now that I am far away and cannot be charged by the local Lobatse elders.

Profession versus tradition

Being a medical doctor and handling both the living and the dead human beings, it was not going to be easy to avoid talking about dying, death and sex. Not an easy thing for any medical doctor or health professional to do. So as expected, I failed to keep the instruction or request, by virtue of my professional training. Can you imagine life without the maternity wards, sexually transmitted infections or venereal diseases' clinics or genito-urinary medicine (GUM) clinics, as they are called in UK? The name "GUM" can be misleading. It has nothing to do with the dental clinics or dentists.

The incident with the elder reminds me of another time, when an aunt of mine came to visit me at the University Teaching Hospital Medical School in Lusaka, Zambia, in the mid 1980s. She ordered me to *"...come home and bath in traditional medicines."* This instruction came after she had heard that I was in the operating theatre conducting evacuations or cleaning out wombs of young female patients who had come into hospital with incomplete abortions or *"...retained products of conception (RPOC)"* as the doctors and nurses would say. These hospital operations were conducted

43

almost daily. So you can imagine the amount of bathing in traditional herbs that one would need to do, if we were to keep and follow tradition.

In many African cultures, an *"abortion"* or *"miscarriage"* is a big issue that needs a lot of rituals for *"cleansing"* the woman who has aborted or has had a miscarriage. One never has sexual intercourse with a woman who has had an abortion, miscarriage or lost, by death, a sexual partner without her being cleansed by the village medicine man or herbalist. There is a belief of many unexplained illnesses, chronic coughs or even death for the men who have sex with such *"unclean"* women. Hospital treatment with pain-killers and antibiotics is not enough. A lady who has aborted has to be cleansed traditionally, in many African communities. The women or relatives might not talk about this tradition, but it is usually done, quietly.

Several families in some African countries have a family traditional doctor just as the English have a family general practitioner commonly known as a GP. The traditional doctor is usually consulted before any major event in life or serious family decision is taken. This is usually done for health related matters, work related issues, body protection from evil spirits, purchase of cars, homes and land. The ancestral spirits have to be consulted and appeased. The purchased personal commodities have to be "cleansed" and blessed with specially treated water or traditional beer.

Equally there are some African countries where many families do not even know a single thing about these tribal traditions or cultures, let alone believe in them. The cultures have been lost or eroded along the years. Many others believe it is "*...rubbish, superstitions or mumbo jumbo."* Some educated colleagues want nothing to do with *"...superstitions...backward African beliefs...black magic!"* Some even believe that traditional doctors are all *"...quacks and a danger to society!"*

Despite these varied views, there are some traditional doctors or herbalists who are very good in what they do. There are also some traditional doctors who hold university degrees in various disciplines. Two of my good friends were traditional doctors. One was a brilliant mathematician lecturing at the university and he also comprehended and articulated the Commonwealth Queen's English language very well and was forever dressed in suits. The other was a humble teacher, teaching chemistry and physics at a local secondary school. These are not the typical stereo-typed traditional doctors that you hear of that are portrayed as half-dressed, wearing masks and surrounded by bones or dancing around a patient by the western media. Some of these traditional doctors are highly schooled men and women with university degrees who can teach the media a point or two.

Some gatekeepers of culture and tradition believe that the influence of the western world has led to the erosion and loss of important African values and that is why *"...infections like HIV infection and AIDS are out of control. We have not adhered to culture and the African way of life.*

Cultures and traditions that kept us in check, morally and spiritually, are unfortunately being slowly eroded by western influence."

The African elders and traditionalists blame the influence of the *"western culture"* through the media and especially the televisions and films for many *"...bad behaviours ...immorality ...unusual sexual practices...mouth on vagina, that is disgusting...eating a penis like a lollipop, that is disgusting...lack of respect..."* in Africa. The tribal leaders believe western influence has led to the development of a sexually *"...lost generation in the youth of today."* Talk to the elders on this subject and you will hear them say, *"...these children have no identity...they do not relate with African upbringings...Which children? These are foreign children...we have lost our children!"*

Barriers to teaching African folks on health matters

One day at my workplace, in London, one of my English colleagues commented on *"...how much we don't know about your folks (Africans)."* This was after two Africans who did not see eye to eye got into a big quarrel that almost ended up physical. I told my English friend, that certain things are hard to understand, unless you live amongst those people. I gave him the example of the United Kingdom and the four countries that make up the United Kingdom – England, Scotland, Ireland and Wales. *"To many an African in Africa, you are one and the same people,"* I said to him. He raised his hand, in protest and complained about how wrong I was. I told him to now think of fifty-four countries in Africa and their people, their beliefs, their religions and their ways of life. He kept quiet. Adult learning had taken place.

HIV infection and AIDS information dissemination has not been easy, as many foreign consultants have learnt the hard way. What are the major barriers or obstacles to sharing or communicating information effectively in the village?

Some barriers or obstacles are:

- **Language.** Note that despite being one country, for example such as Zambia, there are close to 72 languages or dialects in Zambia alone. Botswana has about 16 languages and what of the other 52 countries in Africa? You can see what that means in terms of effective public health messages and communication. Compare that to the United States of America or the United Kingdom where they generally have one or two languages to communicate with or conduct business in.

- **Language translation.** Challenges of translation of medical or technical (jargon) terms into the "normal" everyday vocabulary or languages.

- **Cultures and traditions.** Culture is a way of life. Some of these can be strongly embedded and will take more than faith and prayers to change them. As they say, *"You cannot teach your grandmother how to suckle eggs"* or *"...you can take a horse to the river, but you cannot make it drink the water."*

- **Literacy levels.** Like most countries, Africans have the very educated with three, four or five degrees or postgraduate qualifications and those who have never seen the inside of a classroom. One thing I have realised is that some of the best run HIV infection and AIDS prevention, care and support programmes are run by people who have never seen the four walls of the inside of a classroom. That is the reason that Livingstone and Lobatse paid more attention to the consultants in the name of villagers. The villagers live with HIV infection and AIDS every single day of their lives. It is not only a World AIDS day event.

- **The "brain-drain".** This exodus or migration of doctors, nurses and paramedics for the western world has been a big blow to Africa. These migrating healthcare workers are the backbone of successful programmes in their countries. Unfortunately the skills are being transferred abroad in this global village. Several health facilities in Africa do not have specific healthcare workers that can seriously focus on HIV infection and AIDS alone. There are many other public health programmes that need equal, undivided attention and to be managed equally.

- **"Thinking for the Africans"** if that makes sense. Health officials have a major problem of *"telling"* people what to do instead of consulting and working together with the community folks. It is about *"...them (The ignorant community members) and us (The know it all)."* Mind you Athlone Hospital belonged to the first group, the ignorant community members. I am one of those ignorant villagers. We were usually told what to do from headquarters or by foreign experts. Fortunately we knew what we were *"...wrongly"* doing and therefore never listened to the experts and were rewarded with two documented *"...best practises..."* in Botswana that are being replicated.

- **Economics and poverty levels.** Very controversial area, especially after the South African President was (mis)understood to have said that *"Poverty causes AIDS."* For the records, *"The virus called HIV causes HIV infection. The virus called HIV causes AIDS."* Poverty is one of the many factors that may lead to one becoming infected with HIV. Equally poverty might affect the care and support of people living with HIV infection and AIDS due to the lack of resources. It is a vicious cycle.

- **Political.** You will be surprised at how affiliation to political parties can make or break programmes. How programmes can be supported or not supported. It is sad, that petty (party) politics and personalities disturb well intended projects or programmes that impact on millions of people living with and affected by HIV infection and AIDS. It is life and death that we are talking about. *"Pamodzi (Togetherness)"* and unity is required.

- **Social upbringing.** As they say, *"Charity begins at home."* Unfortunately, for many homes and families they do not talk about sexual matters. Even the schools fail to deliver *"sex education"* as the teachers are *"...too embarrassed to teach on sex, sexuality and relationships!"* It is not easy for many to talk about sexual intercourse.

- **Spiritual and faith beliefs.** It is very sad that there are still a lot of faith communities out there that believe that *"...HIV infection and AIDS are for sinners...for people who are promiscuous...a punishment from God...for pagans...for prostitutes...for people who were doing things that they were not supposed to be doing... so justly reap what you sow!"*

- *"Healing"* **of HIV infection and AIDS.** Some Faith communities believe that they can heal AIDS *"...through the blood and stripes of Jesus... bind the demon of AIDS!"* Some faith communities even stop the clients from taking antiretroviral therapy and tell them to *"...believe in the power of prayer ...power of God...to believe in a miracle...Amen!"* The faith leaders break confidentiality when they mention *"...the sister or brother's name when committing them for special healing!"* Where is the confidentiality?

    Prayers and medicines should be taken together for a positive reaction and a miracle. These same faith community leaders do not stop their congregations from taking diabetes, asthma, hypertension, malaria or arthritis medications. Some of the pastors and ministers are on anti-HIV drugs or antiretroviral therapy. Why stop treatment or drugs for controlling levels of HIV infection in the body and improving the quality of life?

- **Technological reasons.** Note that computers and cell-phones might be there in Africa, but we still have a long way to go to make them accessible to the majority. Whereas South Africa might be more advanced than some European countries, in areas involving the use of computers such as e-commerce and tele-medicine, there are some African countries that are only coming to terms with the introduction of computers as a tool for information dissemination, education, monitoring and communication in a world with HIV infection and AIDS.

- The younger generation understand computers and are growing up with them, but the older generation who are still in key project or programme positions might just have the basic knowledge. Most of Africa still depends on the old time tested traditional methods of teaching and disseminating information, through text-books, leaflets, magazines, posters, the flip-charts and pictures. Computers are not yet part of the normal household furniture of the average home. Pictures and posters have been for quite a time and will do so for quite a while.

All these factors and many others play a role in the lack of or poor development of various intervention strategies for reducing and containing the spread of HIV infection and AIDS. These factors equally affect the care and support of people living with and affected by HIV infection and AIDS. We have some soul searching to do before we lose millions of more souls in the developing countries, as we quibble on whether Pictures in AIDucation is a workable intervention strategy or remains *"...shock tactics do not work!"*

The cover of this book, PICTURES IN AIDUCATION, has twelve of the twenty four pictures that are used to teach on "Basic Facts on HIV infection and AIDS." Are the cover pictures shocking? They are designed in a "C" shape for you to see. *"Seeing is very different from being told."*

HIV infection and AIDS are complex and simple matters

HIV infection and AIDS matters are not only about sex, sexual partners and condoms. HIV infection and AIDS management is both a complex and simple matter. It is a...

- health, political and cultural matter
- communications, behavioural and emotional issue
- pastoral, educational and financial matter
- developmental, legal and ethical issue
- social, security and a humans right issue
- company, workplace and administrative matter.

What has happened in many developing countries in terms of raising HIV infection and AIDS awareness has been massive information dissemination and literature distribution, western style, by the many local healthcare workers and foreign consultants. Well intended foreign programmes for Africa have remained foreign. Ownership has reminded foreign with commands or instructions coming in from Europe or America.

Athlone team introduction at workshops

The Athlone AIDS Awareness team when invited out had several introduction styles. One such introduction was just to show off and impress on the audience the broadness of the social impact of HIV infection and AIDS. The team would spread out and sit amongst the audience, like any other guests. When the chairman or Master of Ceremonies (MC) handed over or called upon the team, the team would enter in style. Each team member would stand up in the audience and mention his or her name. Each would walk down to the front, talking to the audience on the matters or issues listed above as he or she came to sit in front;

"My name is Ronald of the triple A Team. AIDS is about information. It is about receiving information, sharing information or distributing information. Ignorance is no defence. Why should we not know about AIDS when there is so much information around us? Why?"

"My name is Vaja of the Athlone Anti-AIDS Project. AIDS is about health. AIDS is about the WHO definition of health. AIDS is about the physical, social and mental well-being of people. AIDS is about the psychological and emotional well being of man and woman. AIDS is about your health!"

"My name is Nancy and I am a member of the Athlone AIDS Awareness team. AIDS is about sex. AIDS is about family planning and birth. AIDS is about fathers, mothers, uncles, aunts, brothers, sisters and children. AIDS affects all of us. You have a role to play in stopping the spread of AIDS!"

"My name is Proctor. AIDS is about love. AIDS is about compassion. AIDS is about hope. AIDS is about botho (humanity). Remember that a friend with AIDS is still my friend!"

"My name is Phaks, a member of the A-Team. AIDS is about the Church. There is AIDS in the church. AIDS is about the home, the village, the schools, the workplace, the army, the police and the transporters. AIDS is about you and me! AIDS is about Pastoral Care!"

"My name is William, a social worker and member of the Athlone Team. AIDS is about gender issues. AIDS is about violence, rape and irresponsible behaviour. AIDS is about respect for each other."

AIDUCATION

Gentlemen do not rape, do drugs or indulge in risky behaviour that can spread sexually transmitted infections, including HIV infection, from one person to another. We are all responsible for our sexual behaviours. *"Love responsibly!" "Love carefully!"*

HIV stands for Human Immunodeficiency Virus (HIV). The virus called HIV causes AIDS in most men, women and children. HIV infection can be prevented. AIDS can be stopped.

5. DEATH AND DYING

"Death is like a robe that everyone has to wear one day."

African saying

"Good dying and good death"

The increased deaths, suffering and misery in the early 1990s made me ask for an in-service lecture to discuss *"Good Dying and Good Death"* at our weekly Athlone Hospital in-service lectures held on Thursdays. The Athlone Team was not comfortable. This was a very *"...sensitive subject that you are touching ngaka!"* confided one of my team members. It was no surprise when the hospital management team refused permission for the lecture. Reasons given:

- *"Taboo subject"*
- *"Insensitive and inhuman"*
- *"Do not talk about death"*
- *"You will be cursed"*
- *"You will bring negative forces – spirits – on yourself"*
- *"You do not understand our (Botswana) culture"*
- *"It is not African Culture."*

In 1994, Athlone hospital began the long overdue three day AIDucation workshops for the hospital staff of two hundred and fifty workers. The hospital staff included medical doctors, nurses, paramedics, administration staff and general duty staff. No one was left out as HIV infections and AIDS would affect everybody in one way or another. From the Hospital Superintendent to the grounds' men, all were taken away for three days of comprehensive AIDucation each. We were all at risk and therefore we were all responsible for taking positive actions to decrease or prevent new HIV infections. We were all responsible for caring and supporting people already living with and affected by HIV infection and AIDS. We were all being called upon to show the *"ubunthu (humanity)"* in us.

The hospital management team and senior managers were the first to be taken away from the hospital for three whole days to attend the Pictures in AIDucation workshops. Leaders always want to be the first to know about new issues before their subordinates. Many managers do not want to be told about new things by their juniors. This is a fact that is usually over-looked. Armed with that fact, the Athlone team took the senior managers away to a local hotel, Cumberland Hotel, for three days of a social intercourse with HIV infection and AIDS. The hospital managers complained about *"...three days being too long just to discuss AIDS!"* They were further worried about the running of the hospital. They later discovered that three days was too short a time. I must add that the hospital ran better without them.

The *"Cumberland Experience"* away days, proved very successful. The Management Team (Hospital Superintendent, Matron and Administrator), senior nurses and hospital administrators were all AIDucated. A new AIDucation culture was born in Lobatse that would be repeated every year. The managers there after always blessed all our future workshops and gave us tremendous support. Some senior staff initially had been against the Athlone Project and were fighting it. They were *"converted"* after Pictures in AIDucation, which had a total of ninety-six colour pictures on various aspects of HIV infection and AIDS. The pictures talked to the senior staff. *"Seeing is believing and seeing is very different from being told!"* The senior staff listened to the pictures as the pictures talked to them. The senior staff responded positively. There was effective communication through visuals. The visual impact was instant. There was instant feedback. Learning had taken place at management level. The major hurdle had been cleared. The path for AIDucation was clear.

The Lobatse AIDucation Programme

The pictures worked wonders in raising HIV infection and AIDS awareness. Whereas initially the Athlone Project was *"...Mapara's programme"* there was a change of heart in many as the reality of the gravity of the Botswana HIV infection and AIDS situation began to dawn on the citizens. The Athlone Hospital AIDS Awareness Project was no longer *"...Mapara's programme,"* as it became *"...the Lobatse programme"* in the village.

The Batswana have a local saying that says, *"Moja morago ke kgosi* (literally means that *he who eats last is Chief.* Translated to *he who eats at the end is like the Chief)."* The Athlone AIDS Awareness team turned the saying around and made the chiefs eat first. The strategy paid dividends. It worked successfully. During the same year, in 1994, the Hospital Management Team bought two televisions, a video-recorder and a video camera for the Pictures in AIDucation programme. Later on, in the same year, Athlone Hospital received a slide projector from The United Nations Development Programme (UNDP) to use for showing the AIDucation pictures in the awareness raising campaign.

The hospital leadership was committed to see Athlone Hospital's public health programme succeed. With such support, failure was not an option. The project team never even thought of failure. It was not part of their vocabulary. So long as HIV infection and AIDS were in the local community, Athlone Hospital would keep on picturing HIV infection and AIDS for the many years to come. Athlone Hospital would lead and others would follow, locally, nationally and internationally.

51

After the managers were AIDucated, the rest of the Athlone Hospital workers were divided into small groups and taken out for three days each to the local Lobatse community halls, in Peleng and Woodhall locations, where the Athlone Project *"pictured"* HIV infection and AIDS matters. It took almost ten weeks to empower all the 250 hospital workers, but it was worth every single day. The dedication and commitment by the hospital staff was second to none. Athlone Hospital had one spirit and one vision. The future of Botswana was in our hands. AIDucation was in gear.

The hospital workers deferred their leave days, sick off days and holidays during that period. The workers did not want the hospital services to feel their absence - be it clinical, nursing, X-ray, laboratory, pharmacy, dispensary, supplies, social work, catering, gardening, grounds, security, laundry, tailoring, transport, administration, switch-board, medical records or the mortuary services. It was very touching to be part of such a humanitarian initiative and a powerful hospital, Athlone Hospital. The resistance to the *status quo* was finally crumbling as the matron, with a smile of satisfaction said, *"Athlone Hospital AIDS Awareness Project has finally arrived!"*

Dying and death

In the AIDucation workshops *"Good Dying and Good Death"* was tactfully introduced after the hospital workers saw, in pictures, the various economical, social, emotional, clinical and physical presentations or manifestations of HIV infection and AIDS. The prediction of the impending deaths to come, not that might come, but will definitely come was the beginning of the discussion, finally, of *"Good Dying and Good Death."* This was done through ninety-six pictures and several videos. There was active participation and fruitful discussions on the subject of death and dying. Barriers were finally broken. Athlone Hospital was talking death and dying. The Athlone team asked the workshop participants what they understood by *"Good Dying and Good Death."*

The answers included:

- *"Pain free death"*
- *"Peaceful death"*
- *"Control of troublesome and embarrassing symptoms like chronic diarrhoea"*
- *"Depart having solved financial problems: debts owing, school fees and future school arrangement for children"*
- *"To die before I become bed-ridden or a burden to my relatives"*
- *"Secure accommodation for my family"*
- *"Wish to die at home amongst family members"*
- *"Do not prolong my suffering with drips to keep me alive"*

- *"For God to forgive our nation"*
- *"Support from community for my funeral"*
- *"To die peacefully in my sleep"*
- *"The last happy farewell"*
- *"To die without pain"*
- *"For others to learn about AIDS from my suffering and death"*
- *"To mention at my burial that I died of AIDS and not a long illness"*
- *"Not to cry at my funeral, but to celebrate my life on this earth with music and dance"*
- *"Having a responsible relative or friend to look after my children when I die"*
- *"To die looking beautiful while my hair is still black"*
- *"Not to waste money on my funeral, but to give the money to my wife and children"*
- *"To be at peace with my creator, Jehovah"*
- *"To know that your team (Athlone AIDS Awareness Project) will save as many people as possible and will never give up."*

It took *"picturing"* HIV infections and AIDS to finally discuss *"good dying and good death"* with the Lobatse community. *"Seeing is believing"* say the English and the Kenyans say, *"Seeing is very different from being told."*

One workshop participant summed up what *"good dying and good death"* was by talking about his mother who had died of old age, may her soul rest in peace. The participant glowed and said,

"My mother lived and enjoyed life to the fullest. She died a peaceful death in her sleep. She never suffered, she was never in pain. The whole village was there at her burial and the choirs sang heavenly songs, while the angels looked down.

She had an excellent funeral and a good send off!

Man, I have got no complaints.

Amen, amen and amen! "

AIDucation Away Days

Those AIDucation workshops were the beginning of many more of such two to three days workshops out of the hospital, annually, with the whole hospital staff of two hundred and fifty, over the next ten years. Effective community AIDucation needs days and not an hour or two. AIDucation should not be rushed. For Athlone Hospital, taking the entire staff away for two to three days to discuss various aspects of HIV infection and AIDS became a norm. Lobatse Mental Hospital (LMH), The Institute of Health Sciences (IHS), Lobatse Town Council and Good-Hope Primary Hospital would send down their staff to join the Athlone family in AIDucation. Athlone Hospital held similar Pictures in AIDucation workshops on:-

- o Clinical presentations or signs and symptoms of HIV infection and AIDS
- o Tuberculosis and AIDS
- o Home based care
- o Counselling
- o Pastoral Care and "The Good Samaritan"
- o Orphans and other vulnerable children
- o Prevention of Parent to Child Transmission of HIV infection
- o Provision of Antiretroviral Therapy in Botswana.

Letting the tears flow freely

Apart from imparting knowledge and getting each other AIDucated, these workshops were therapeutic in their own ways, as members of staff spoke freely of their personal losses (deaths) and hardships that were a result of HIV infection and AIDS touching their families. They shared their painful experiences with each other. For many, they finally grieved as the bottled up, delayed, bereavement of past years began to pour out. It took Pictures in AIDucation to release the bottled emotions of sorrow. It took AIDucation to admit that AIDS had visited the family. That AIDS had taken a member of the family.

There was one AIDucation workshop where almost the whole group of twenty five participants broke down and wept as one after the other related how HIV infection and AIDS had touched the home or the family. How AIDS had wrecked the family. How AIDS had created orphans. How AIDS had caused misery. How AIDS had caused suffering and poverty. How AIDS had affected the faith of Christians as they asked God questions, that He only can answer.

It was heart-breaking, depressing and at the same time comforting, if that makes sense. People had been bottled up for too long and were slowly opening up. Some had not grieved and were only now beginning to grieve and to come to terms with the reality of HIV infection and AIDS. It was not the perceived witchcraft *"...by jealous relatives or neighbours."* Some even related the clinical pictures of tuberculosis (TB), Kaposi's sarcoma, herpes zoster and skin rashes to the deceased or departed. Many believed that their relatives died of AIDS, but were not sure as, *"...nobody in the family talked about it."* One participant, who had lost an elder sister three years earlier, said that she had *"...suspected that it was AIDS. Now I know it was AIDS. She died in pain. We buried her three year old baby a month ago."* The participant could not contain her emotions. She broke down and cried uncontrollably. We paused in respect, with heads bowed, as other participants sobbed silently in support and sang a hymn. Were the other participants crying because of her losses or was it due to their own hidden pains and losses that the tears trickled down?

Indirectly Athlone Hospital was removing stigmatisation and normalising HIV infection and AIDS. I remember some of my patients joking in front of their relatives about death just before they died as they said, *"I learnt too late, kadoyo (small insect) has clobbered me...The day you will leave Botswana Chipolopolo (Zambia national football team) will be beaten by the Zebras (Botswana national football team)...this little bug knows no boundaries...My wife and baby gone. Now it is me...Sala sentle, Ngaka (Stay well, Doctor)...talk to the children. Sex was good before AIDS. Now it is a life or death activity...that penis in the vagina could be the beginning of things!"*

Some dying clients wished the Athlone team well *"...in your fight with AIDS. Never give up!"* The *"...never give up"* became Athlone's rallying cry when things got rough. Even as I write this sentence, my eyes have become misty as I see the faces of all those fallen great men and women who were our patients, clients and friends. Some travelled from hundreds of miles away just to talk about their health to *"...a doctor who understands AIDS"* before the various counselling and emotional support services were put in place. I was a pillar of strength to many lonely, stigmatised and isolated clients living with HIV infection and AIDS.

There was a period when I asked Botswana Telecommunications (BTC) to *"...remove Dr Edwin Mapara's home telephone number"* in the Botswana telephone directory. This was because of the constant phone calls coming in, at home after hours, in the evening. Due to unforeseen circumstances and lack of counselling services in the early 1990s, I began running unplanned HIV infection counselling sessions on the telephone. It was not easy to say *"No!"* to the many people living with HIV infection or AIDS who wanted to talk to me from across the country. I even had one client that phoned from a village almost eight hundred miles away. It was a difficult decision, but BTC understood my dilemma and helped me out by removing my name from the telephone directory.

As part of stress management and managing burn-out, I used to tell the team to, *"... leave HIV infection and AIDS in the hospital when you go home. Home and after hours is for the family."* This also applied to me, although I must admit it was difficult. Occasional AIDucation related phone calls came through and a few clients came home to see me.

Coincidentally, "Chipolopolo" was beaten by the Zebras, when I left Botswana. That was something that I do not remember happening before. I thought of *"the departed"* when that happened and I think the departed must have smiled in their sleep.

Messages from beyond the graves

Many of my clients died of AIDS and I received the sad news, at times many weeks after the burial. I can still see some of those darling grandmothers and mothers bringing me the sad news of death. To many HIV affected families I was their *"son"* and part of the family. The messages weakened me and strengthened me at the same time. Those messages depressed me and at the same time motivated me to continue. There were times I was so exhausted, burnt out and thought of giving up, but voices would tell me to *"...continue..."* coming from beyond the graves. Those messages were echoed by the relatives of the dead who kept and honoured the last wishes of their patients and travelled many miles to come to deliver those messages to me. Most of those messages were of gratitude and well wishes such as *"...thank you...continue...do not give up...Modimo oteng (God is there)."*

For others, I received the messages at the funeral houses of the burials I attended as I was part of the family in many house-holds. The messages that were delivered were, *"...Ngaka (Doctor), your patient is no more, we buried her a few weeks ago...Ngaka (Doctor), she sent her love and she said thank you for treating her like a human being...May you see many wonderful days ahead...she said do not forget her, you were her best friend...He said 'yebo' (thank you) and "...Zambia (Dr Mapara's nickname) keep showing those pictures...God be with you...do not leave our children to die of AIDS, talk to them...Your name, Maparapara (In between the legs), suits you and your calling."*

There was one Saturday, when I travelled with the Athlone team to the village of Mahalapye to attend a funeral. On the day of the burial, I was shocked to see at the entrance of the graveyard, amongst the freshly dug graves, a tombstone with a name of one of my closest female clients. She had died about two months ago. That seriously jolted me. My heart ached. There was that heartache that one experiences, when told about sudden bad news. I stopped with some team members to pay our last respects to her, before proceeding to bury our other friend. *"Robala ka kagiso tsala"* - Sleep in peace my friend.

Each death took a piece of me. Talk of a broken heart, mine was a shattered heart. I was never trained to take in so much suffering and death. I literally looked at death in the eyes of my clients almost every week. I had to cope and manage in the best way I knew. How? Continue with AIDucation and forming support groups. I refused to accept defeat or to lose to AIDS. This was a personal battle. There was no surrendering. The battle continues. *"Aluta continua!"*

The Athlone Hospital Burial Society

It was from the Athlone Hospital AIDucation workshops, that another *"best practice"* initiative was born, the Athlone Hospital Burial Society. It was an idea brought up by the Industrial Class (unskilled staff), not the doctors or nurses (skilled staff). The Athlone burial society was created to help alleviate the suffering of hospital workers during bereavements and to reduce the burden brought about by death in the immediate family. For many healthcare workers at Athlone Hospital, the major concern was the financial burden caused by the death of a family member. Hospital workers made monthly contributions to a fund that would help each member in case of a death or bereavement in the immediate family. This money was a *"...welcome financial gesture"* and a relief to many families when a death occurred in the family. Small as it may sound, Pula 500 (£100) in those days, was a lot of money. This amount would be the initial money handed out, to the family, to help out with the costs of the funeral, while other donations and contributions were being collected, which could amount to P2000 (£400) or more.

The financial costs of a funeral can be heavy in Africa. There is the cost of the food and drinks, to feed the hundreds of guests. There are the burial and celebration costs. There are travel and transport costs for relatives coming in from the rural areas. There are costs for the coffin and the tombstone. There are costs, in some cases, of having to transport bodies back to their villages of birth within Botswana or countries of origin. AIDS has dictated and shaped many old and new social programmes in Africa. Burial societies are some of the off-shoots of AIDS in Africa. It is like having a life insurance cover or life policy.

Whoever imagined that the once local, Lobatse, controversial, emotional *"death and dying"* lecture or talk in Lobatse would be part of the making of national burial societies across Botswana. This reminds me of my medical school days, when I attended my first post-mortem in the mortuary at the University Teaching Hospital. There was a bold worded inscription over the entrance door to the post-mortem room that read, *"This is where death delights to save the living."*

African funerals and burials

Talking about death and dying, I have attended more than a hundred and fifty funerals and burials in Zambia and Botswana. Funerals and burials in Africa are conducted very differently from those in Europe.

- Dying patients prefer to be nursed at home or the village, mostly by elderly care-givers in the home based care programme.

- Some patients know that they are dying and prepare for death, with the Bible by their bedside. They give their last instructions on earth to family members by the bedside, before they shut their eyes for the final sleep.
- Death is a community event and many community members play a role:
  - The church choirs take turns to sing at the funeral house, in the evenings, especially if the deceased was a member of a faith community.
  - The soldiers, police and prisoners help in providing and putting up tents for the mourners. They also provide fire wood for the fire(s) that burn all day and all night at the funeral gatherings, until after the burial, when the fires are put out and the yards are swept clean.
  - The community contributes towards the purchase of or providing food and drinks
  - The community members play various roles to ease the burden of the bereaved families, by cooking, cleaning up and doing other household chores.
  - The traditional leaders, local Members of Parliament and politicians are usually present as they are the elected *"...servants of the people"* who represent government.
- Traditional rituals are performed and prayers are held while washing and dressing the corpse.
- Women mourn alone in the house or at the back of the house, sitted on the floor. Men mourn under the tent or veranda, at the front of the house, sitted on chairs, traditional stools or logs that have been placed like benches.
- Women in Zambia traditionally wear a "chitenge (wrapper)" that is wrapped around the waist and completely covers the legs and a black head scarf that covers the hair. In Botswana a scarf or shawl over the shoulders is a must for the women attending a funeral.
- Men in Zambia dress in casual clothes, while in Botswana, a jersey, jacket or coat must be worn on top of the shirt. Black or dark coloured clothes are observed in both countries.
- Night vigils are observed in both countries.
- In Zambia, wailing by the women is common at funeral homes in support of the grieving widow or to announce the arrival of new mourners. Men tend to be silent and walk in quietly.
- In Botswana and South Africa mourning is generally a silent affair. The nationals do not wail or are not as *"...dramatic"* as the Zambians or Zimbabweans.
- Body viewing or paying of last respects is done at the church, funeral parlour or graveyard, in Zambia. In Botswana, the body viewing is done at the house of the deceased in the early morning hours. The coffin, with the body inside it, spends the last night in the house of the deceased in the bedroom or main room.

- The church service in Zambia is conducted at the graveyard, while in Botswana it is held at the home of the deceased and with a short service at the graveyard.

- When the coffin is lowered in the grave, the immediate family members are the first to throw in soil to cover the coffin. The extended family, invited guests and senior citizens follow to throw in soil. Afterwards the men usually line up to take turns in shovelling in soil to fill the grave. The spade or shovels are picked up from the ground and used. One is not supposed to hand the shovel or spade to another man. It must be picked up from the ground. With the changing roles of community members, women are now seen shovelling soil into the graves, something that was never seen before AIDS came on the scene.

- After the burial, the mourners are supposed to go back to the funeral house, wash their hands at the entrance of the yard and partake in the meals and drinks that are served. This is very important. Not taking part in eating the meal(s) served can be grossly misunderstood and misinterpreted. You do not want to make that mistake. Believe you me, eat with the mourners.

- Traditional talks take place led by an elderly family spokesman. The mourners are thanked for their support and dispersed with a plea of *"...not to forget to look after the bereaved family"* especially where the bread-winner has died.

- Depending on the cultures, immediate bereaved family members have a hair-cut. In other communities, women dress in black for a certain period or have a black piece of cloth on their shoulder on their dressing to show that they are in a period of mourning.

- Recently another culture of *"After tears party"* has been introduced. This is a happy (party) event held in the evening after the burial, to celebrate the life of the deceased or the departed. This trend started in South Africa and is now catching on in Botswana. In the early days there were some mixed feelings about mourning in the morning and partying in the evening.

AIDUCATION

Immune or body defence ("soldiers") system can be improved by *"living positively"* with HIV infection or AIDS. That means good nutrition, adequate exercise, having plenty of rest, no smoking and no drinking alcohol, avoid stress and always use condoms when having sexual intercourse.

Judgemental attitudes should not be encouraged. These negative attitudes lead to stigma, isolation and discrimination of people living with HIV infection or AIDS. Judge not, lest you be judged.

6. PICTURES IN AIDUCATION

"Great events may stem from words of no importance."

African saying

Missing link in health talks

Experience had taught us at Livingstone General Hospital, Zambia and Athlone Hospital, Botswana, that the missing link in talking about sexually transmitted infections was the lack of picturing sexually transmitted infections including HIV infection and AIDS to the many "picturate" community members and communities. The lack of imagination in making HIV infection and AIDS visible has been man's downfall. The selfishness of healthcare workers with their medical illustrations, colour clinical images or pictures has played a major role in the spread of HIV infection and AIDS.

Hospitals in Africa have shifted into the homes, but the medical illustration units or libraries have remained behind in the hospital. So the caregivers or relatives see their herpes zoster, Kaposi's sarcoma, cervical cancer, non-healing wounds, severe rashes and gross bedsores on their patients in their homes and wonder what these things are. The care-givers were never taught about these things. In some cases the doctor or the nurse made a genuine effort and explained to the relatives who listened, but did not hear, that this is a *"...varicella zoster rash...human herpes virus type 8...human papilloma virus (HPV)...depletion of the B and T cells...natural killer cells have been destroyed...!"* Jargon, jargon and more jargon.

For pictures' sake, simplicity and clarity why not sit down with the relatives and show them these pictures and explain to them what is happening to their patient and what to expect as the disease progresses. Prepare the relatives or care-givers mentally for the inevitable, for death, if the conditions worsen. Many people will thank you for it. Without the anti-HIV drugs in the towns and villages of Africa, the communities will see more and more of these types of conditions, not seen in Europe and America, where the antiretroviral therapy have improved the quality of life of people living with HIV infection and AIDS. It is a fact that in Africa and Asia AIDS is still fatal, while in Europe and America AIDS is a chronic manageable disease.

It is a fact that almost 90% of the world's HIV infections and AIDS patients are in the developing countries, while 10% live in the developed world. Meanwhile 90% of the world's anti-HIV or anti-AIDS drugs are found in the developed world and less than 10% of these drugs are in the developing countries. So the sooner the African communities get used to seeing these various clinical presentations of the infections and diseases, through Pictures in AIDucation, the better for their patients and for themselves, so as to take the necessary care and precautions.

It is not uncommon to discharge AIDS patients for home-based care in the daytime only to have them re-admitted at night through Accident and Emergency or the Casualty Department. The relatives *"...disappear...vanish..."* but keep an ear to the ground waiting to hear that the patient has died. Some families even travel hundreds of miles away to go and leave the patient in a far away hospital or health facility for the fear of nursing some of the cancers, especially Kaposi's sarcoma that can be visibly frightening, even to the strong and hard-hearted.

Severe Kaposi's sarcoma (KS) patients are not easy to manage at home and the offensive smell of KS does not make it any easier. I know of families where the children were sent away to live with other relatives until the patient(s) died. In other cases, patients had small traditional huts built for them so that *"... he does not frighten the others..."* in the two bed-roomed house that had a total of five occupants or more, which is not uncommon in the developing countries.

If the African leadership will wait for the foreign consultants to come and tell us what to do, then we have a very long wait. Meanwhile HIV infection and AIDS will not wait. The two public health disasters will continue to reap in abundance. As the Bible says, *"My people die due to lack of Knowledge."* A number of the contracted foreign consultants have never even seen some of these conditions that HIV infection and AIDS presents with. That means that the international consultants will have to be taught about these conditions by the local doctors in Africa and then the consultants will teach the local people. What an expensive round about way of conducting business.

Africa has to believe in itself. African leaders have to believe in their professionals. Africans must be proactive and aggressive in preventing new HIV infections. There is an African saying that says, *"When you have learnt, you must teach others."* Unfortunately a lot of the *"brain-drain"* doctors could not teach, as the local leadership did not believe in them.

I no longer get surprised when some of the medical doctors in London tell me that they have never seen a TB patient or a patient with herpes zoster or Kaposi's sarcoma during my AIDucation lectures in London. You cannot blame or fault them. With most of the London HIV patients on antiretroviral therapy conditions such as Kaposi's sarcoma will be very rare. I always remember one colleague, who asked me, *"Are you sure it was Kaposi's sarcoma you saw?"* "Loso legolo ki ditseko! (literal translation is *'big death is laughter'*)" meaning you do not know whether to laugh or to cry at the event, happening or the question as in this case." For somebody who was seeing two to three clients of Kaposi's sarcoma on average per month in the later years, this question needed a lecture, which I naturally gave, from the finger-tips.

As for tuberculosis (TB), that is a different story that we will keep for the second book, as the tuberculosis cases increase by the year in the United Kingdom. TB in England will increase by the thousands before getting better. The TB cases are still to rise due to many factors, including homelessness, overcrowding, rampant drug abuse, selective BCG vaccinations and suppressed immunity that could be due to HIV infection. It is a known fact that with HIV infection and AIDS on the increase, the number of TB patients will increase.

A rule of thumb from Athlone Hospital, Botswana, *"...Where there is HIV infection, suspect TB. Where there is TB suspect HIV infection."* TB and HIV infection are related in many countries. An increase in TB cases can be an indicator of increased HIV infections in the community.

The beginning of Pictures in AIDucation

It all began one hot summer day in 1992, in a small village in Lobatse, Botswana, that has a population of about 36, 000 people. Lobatse is famous for its beef industry, the Botswana Meat Commission (BMC). Lobatse is home to the internationally known tinned ECCO beef. Lobatse is also home to Athlone "Teaching" District Hospital, the Lobatse Mental Hospital, the Institute of Health Sciences (IHS) and the High Court of Botswana. By Botswana standards Lobatse is more of a town than a village and has developed around the meat industry. Lobatse was once the capital city of Botswana, before the present capital city called Gaborone.

On that hot summer day, some students from a local secondary school came to Athlone Hospital wanting *"... to see an AIDS patient...so that we can believe that there is AIDS... it is not just a government story to discourage teenage pregnancy."* The boys seriously believed that **AIDS** was *"... an American Ideology for Discouraging Sex!"* Others have said AIDS is **"...an Adults Ideology to Discourage Sex!"** To these young men and many others HIV infection and AIDS were *"invisible!"* It called upon great imagination to picture this *"...new disease."* If anything rumours had it that AIDS was for the *"...bazungu (Europeans)...makgoa (white people)...those who indulge in matanyola (homosexual) activities...as usual the white people blaming Africans for bad things..."* The list can go on and on. These rumours were definitely not true. HIV infection and AIDS affects everybody, whether homosexual, bisexual or "straight" heterosexual. It knows no continent, whether Africa, Asia, America, Australia or Europe. It knows no colour, whether white, black or brown, we are all at risk with HIV infection and AIDS. It favours no religion.

Athlone Hospital could not breach confidentiality and the right of privacy of the patients and clients, to prove that HIV infection and AIDS was real. It was a challenge. Athlone Hospital was in a dilemma. I had to think fast with these youngsters challenging me. The boys had to be convinced about the reality of the situation. It was a window of opportunity not to be missed. I thought of one possible solution, the AIDucation pictures. Arrangements with the students for the next possible option, to show them clinical pictures (medical illustrations), of possible African people living with HIV infection and AIDS was made. The pictures or colour slides to be used were part of the Athlone Hospital audio-visual library, made by Teaching aids At Low Cost, St Albans, United Kingdom for training healthcare workers.

The boys were advised to go back to school and make arrangements with their teachers, for Athlone Hospital staff to go over to talk to them in the near future on HIV infection and AIDS. The boys went back to school very excited. On the same day, in the afternoon, the headmaster of the local secondary school telephoned me. He asked me what I had arranged with his students, as he had never seen them *"...so serious before"* for any activity. He said, *"The boys have arranged a classroom for your lecture on AIDS, this evening. They say that you are coming with some pictures."*

I was stunned and surprised because we had not concluded on a date and the time with the students. In fact the arrangements should have been made through their teacher, headmaster or school administration. I explained to the headmaster what had taken place in the morning when the boys had come over to the hospital. The headmaster and I agreed that since the boys had already prepared the venue and were ready, I would go over at 6.00 pm, after their dinner, to give them a talk on HIV infection and AIDS. The aim of the talk was to prove that AIDS was real.

That same evening in 1992, at 6.00 pm, I arrived at the local school as arranged. Little did I realise at that time, that these young, curious men, had initiated what was to become an international HIV infection and AIDS awareness raising intervention strategy. The AIDucation strategy was going to go local, national and international. It was going to be a global brand. Lobatse was about to write history that evening, that others would be AIDucated from globally.

The headmaster welcomed me and introduced me to the students, who knew me as *"The AIDS Doctor"* from Zambia. The headmaster then left the classroom, so as to give the boys freedom and space with me. The AIDucation lecture of twenty-four colour pictures that was scheduled for one hour, took close to three hours. The clinical pictures were literally *"talking"* to the young men. We had a fruitful, mature dialogue and discussion on sex, relationships and sexually transmitted infections, including HIV infection and AIDS. The students asked all their questions. I answered all their questions. It was like an oral medical examination, from the medical school days, only that this time it was the youth asking me the questions generated from the pictures, and not those mean consultants at medical school towering over me. We covered more ground with the youngsters than we would have covered had I gone with a written handout that had no pictures.

There was effective communication on the subject of HIV infection and AIDS. The feedback was instant. The feedback was very positive. The denial and doubts were removed. HIV infection and

AIDS had become real over night. AIDS had become visible. Behaviour change communication had begun through teaching with colour clinical images or pictures made for teaching healthcare workers. Those over charged, testosterone filled, young men had put me through a tread meal. They had made me see the other side of those medical pictures that had never ever dawned on me, the grassroots side of the AIDucation pictures. Let the pictures talk. The pictures had spoken. The *"picturate"* had heard.

Safer and delayed sex was no longer an option, it was THE option, after the pictures were shown that it was a serious *"...do or die"* matter in the prevention of sexually transmitted infections. *"Seeing is very different from being told!"* That night the African saying was proved very true. It was simply a fantastic dialogue. I did not have to take the boys for a tour in the hospital to show them patients living with HIV infection or AIDS. *"Pictures in AIDucation"* was the *"missing link"* and it had taken the place of that hospital tour request.

AIDucation was born in Lobatse because of a few curious, sexually inquisitive lads. It was the Lobatse community through the boys that initiated Pictures in AIDucation, in Botswana. AIDucation was not initiated by the local scientists, doctors, nurses or foreign consultants. It was sparked by the indigenous young natives. The youth of Lobatse deserve kudos.

Assumptions and attitudes

As healthcare workers, there is so much that we take for granted or assume of the general public, our patients and clients. The general public are more intelligent than we tend to think and admit. That night the students learnt from me and I learnt from them. They listened to me and I listened to them. Effective learning had definitely taken place, both ways. The AIDucation pictures were the *"missing link"* to our community sceptics, cynics and doubters. A new chapter was written in Lobatse through the social intercourse with the students that night. HIV infections and AIDS had become real. HIV infections and AIDS had become visible. HIV infections and AIDS were with us in Lobatse that night. **AIDS** was no longer or joke or an *"American Ideology for Discouraging Sex."* AIDS had become a serious public health problem called in full, *"Acquired Immune Deficiency Syndrome."*

The lesson I took away from the session with the lads was NEVER ever talk, teach or share experiences again on sexually transmitted infections without pictures, to tell the story. Certain things are best described, taught and shared with pictures. After all it has already been said that, *"...a picture is worth a thousand words!"* I used twenty-four pictures that night. The doubting students, who had given me a suspicious look in the morning, had transformed within eight hours, to become staunch, serious believers and AIDucators that night. After *"seeing"* in the night they nodded to the reality and the gravity of the situation in Botswana. *"Seeing is very different from being told!"*

Since 1992, after that classroom session, I have never given a lecture, talk or presentation on HIV infection and AIDS without the AIDucation pictures. The same can be said for the Athlone AIDS Awareness Project Team comprised of nurses and social workers. The nurses and social workers share experiences with the same AIDcation pictures. The Athlone AIDS Awareness Project team and the AIDucation pictures have been inseparable since 1992. The day you hear that Edwin Mapara, in London, or the Athlone Hospital staff in Botswana were giving a talk on AIDS without the colour pictures, you can rest be assured that it was not so. They cannot talk without pictures. I would be totally naked without the pictures. In fact the last time I talked on HIV infection or AIDS without the pictures was before I met those lively high school students in 1992. Those Lobatse students are the unsung heroes of Botswana.

The AIDucation pictures have left their positive impact in many communities and with many individuals. As one lady at one time told me, *"When I see you, I see those pictures and like I told you, never ever again without a condom!"* At least she was better or politer than the lady who said, *"When I see you, I see sex and those pictures!"*

There was also one man who had been locally AIDucated that came to the hospital to give his gratitude for the acquired AIDucation knowledge. He was so excited that he came to the Athlone Hospital out-patient department looking for me so as to thank me for *"...saving my life!"* He caused a scene at the out-patient department, in front of forty or so patients waiting to be seen or consulted by the medical doctors. He told the nurses that he was not a patient, but had to see *"...the AIDS' doctor for having saved my life!"* The nurse reluctantly brought him to the consulting room where I was attending to patients, believing that he wanted to jump the line or queue of patients waiting to see the doctors.

When he saw me, he excitedly shook my hand with a lot of energy and power, repeatedly saying, *"Keitumetsi! Keitumetsi! (Thank you! Thank you!)"* I finally calmed him down and asked him to explain himself, as I could not remember him from the out-patient department or as an in patient on the wards. He answered excitedly, *"Last night I had a few drinks (beer) with this woman at a bar. After the drinks we went to her place. Luckily for me, the light was on when she was undressing. I sobered straight away when I saw that "belt (herpes zoster scar)" on her right side of the chest and under the right breast. I remembered you and those pictures you showed us. Ngaka (doctor) I ran for my life!"*

"Seeing is believing," and *"seeing is very different from being told."* The pictures are very essential in HIV infection or AIDS education (AIDucation).

What is Pictures in AIDucation?

In a nutshell, it is HIV infection and AIDS education (AIDucation) taught with the aid of colour images or pictures in the community. Initially, in 1992, it was simply the use of the clinical AIDucation colour slides, but along the years Athlone Hospital added relevant non-clinical pictures and audio-visual tapes. Local, country, video tapes have made a great impact and bring the message closer to home. The familiar surroundings, language and social life seen in the videos create an *"enabling environment"* to discuss HIV infection and AIDS in the village. AIDS ceases to be a *"...the foreigners' disease."* AIDS becomes our problem. AIDS becomes my problem.

"Pictures in AIDucation" is about;

- making HIV infection and AIDS visible to the public
- stimulating dialogue, making people open up and talk freely on sexual matters
- listening to community members telling YOU (the teacher or facilitator) about what THEY see in the pictures. It is from THEIR information, usually lack of information, that YOU build up your discussion, dialogue, debate or deliverable messages
- local ownership of the AIDucation programmes by the community members
- empowering individuals to run their own community programmes. The village folks should be able to say at the end of the day that, *"We did it by ourselves!"*

It is fascinating what you learn from the general public on the pictures of sexually transmitted infections such as syphilis, gonorrhoea, chancroid, candida (thrush), genital warts and herpes simplex.

Traditional beliefs or stories about the causes of herpes zoster, Kaposi's sarcoma and TB lymphadenopathy or swelling of the lymph nodes are amazing. The local beliefs of causes of illness or disease, traditional treatments and remedies are fascinating in their own ways.

AIDucation is about making HIV infection and AIDS visible and real. It is about making a complicated subject easy. It is about the de-medicalisation of HIV infection and AIDS, which has been too medicalised or hospitalised by the healthcare workers. The Athlone AIDucation pictures used in the discussions included:

- Sexually transmitted infections
- Basic facts on HIV transmission, prevention and care
- Clinical manifestations of HIV infection and AIDS
- HIV prevention and counselling
- Prevention of Parent to Child Transmission (PTCT) of HIV infection.

The video tapes watched or viewed included:

- Born in Africa (Philly Lutaaya)
- TASO: Counselling
- Morehouse : Taking it home; Stigmatisation; Arrogance of High Achievers
- No Need To Blame
- Remember Mpho
- The Bobirwa Home based care programme
- Challenges in Counselling
- The Orphans' Generation and *"What Can I Do?"*

Pictures are not only *"...worth a thousand words"* - they tell *"...the African* story" on HIV infection and AIDS from a cultural point of view. The twenty – four TALC slides are therefore worth 24,000 words. In Africa, communication is all about culture and culture is all about communication. To make or break a programme will depend on working with first and fore-most traditional leaders and the faith community leaders. They hold the cultural, spiritual, and moral values of the village. The healthcare workers are further down the line of responsibility.

Target audience for Pictures in AIDucation

The AIDucation target audience in Botswana was, to put it simply, *"everybody"* in Botswana. Since 1992, some of the audiences or participants in the AIDucation workshops included scientists, people living with HIV infection and AIDS, nurses, paramedics, doctors, social workers, nutritionists, health promoters, dieticians, faith community leaders, pastors, deacons, church elders, church congregations, community village committee members, community associations, transporters, prisoners, teachers and students (primary, secondary, college and university), scouts and girl guides, out of school youths, commercial sex workers (prostitutes), lecturers, journalists, traditional doctors and herbalists, traditional birth attendants, the police, the army, trade unions, civil servants, non-governmental organisations, policy-makers, programme managers, heads of departments, politicians and HIV infection and AIDS consultants, both local and foreign.

In Europe, since August 2002, some of the audiences have been Black and Minority Ethnic (BME) organisations and communities, university students (University of London, Thames Valley University and Cambridge University), teachers, nurses, medical students, doctors, faith communities, health promoters and eight High Commissioners from Africa who are based in London.

The "icing on the cake" for Pictures in AIDucation was my being invited as a Special Guest Speaker at World Health Organisation (WHO), Geneva, Switzerland on World AIDS Day 2004. This was followed by an AIDucation workshop for the AIDS experts on the 2nd December 2004.

The invitation to WHO, Geneva, was facilitated by Ms Emily Bell, who is not a doctor or nurse, whom I met while studying in London. I shared my experiences with her of using Pictures in AIDucation. She later went on to do an internship at WHO, Geneva and invited me over through her department in Geneva, believing I had *"...something special"* to offer in AIDucation.

For once, in almost 20 years of AIDucation, I thought that I would be torn apart by the WHO team of experts on this AIDucation teaching method, as other consultants had said, *"...controversial intervention strategy of using pictures... shock tactics...it has never worked before."* Strangely enough, there was no storm that I had anticipated, all was calm and well. *"The butterflies will fly in formation"* Anne Francis, a motivational speaker, business coach and friend from Norwich would say, when I confided in her about being uncomfortable and having *"...butterflies in my stomach!"*

The positive response and comments by the WHO experts was motivating for lack of a better English word. I even met one of the medical doctors, who had taken part in making some of the AIDucation slides or pictures at WHO Geneva. He was one of the participants in the Pictures in AIDucation session that I held. He was very amused and commented at the end of the session saying that, *"...I never thought that one day I will be taught on HIV infection and AIDS, by my junior, using my own slides of 1989!"* Who can be better placed than that doctor, the author of some of the AIDucation pictures to rate the *"controversial"* Pictures in AIDucation strategy from Botswana?

One of the other WHO experts asked me if Athlone Hospital had ever used the AIDucation strategy on the deaf people, as *"...they (the deaf) use their eyes for communication."* It was embarrassing that here I was an advocate for visuals and yet I had not thought of the deaf who visualised everything. I confessed to her that it had never even dawned on the Athlone Team to address the deaf. She went on to say that she would love her sign language staff *"...to use these visuals to teach the deaf on AIDS."* Another missed opportunity in AIDucation.

AIDUCATION

Knowledge is power. AIDS education (AIDucation) should be shared with as many people as possible. Be generous with your AIDucation. Share the AIDucation with other people around you.

Love must not be lost because someone is living with HIV infection or AIDS. Remember that, *"A friend with HIV infection or AIDS is still my friend!"*

7. RESPONSES, OUTCOMES AND COMMENTS

"One who enters the forest does not listen to the breaking of the twigs in the bush."

African saying

Responses to Pictures in AIDucation at national level

History is repeating itself in the United Kingdom. Folks in the London community are asking me that "old" simple but difficult question again on why other doctors are not teaching with Pictures in AIDucation. Strangely enough, some colleagues at the same AIDucation workshop, seminar or conference platform refer to my pictures when they are talking on their various topics that do not have pictures. To me, that is an indirect way of telling us, in the audience, that their presentations would be much better off, better understood, more empowering and more engaging with colour pictures.

The great reggae musician, Jimmy Cliff, sung about *"Actions speak louder than words!"* In this global, grave public health situation that HIV infection and AIDS dictates we must add that, *"Pictures speak louder than words!"*

I am now sharing my AIDucation pictures with other doctors and health promoters in London. This used to happen in Botswana occasionally, where fellow medical doctors would come and ask for the AIDucation pictures from Athlone Hospital, to help them run workshops in the community over weekends. People wanted to *"...see..."* HIV infection and AIDS but many a healthcare worker has ended up giving the people a lot of jargon that made it no better. There was even one colleague in London, who initially spoke against Pictures in AIDucation, but later used six of the AIDucation pictures to make a point on his presentation on *"Mother to child transmission of HIV infection."* I reminded him of his earlier comments about *"...shock tactics..."* and asked him why he was using *"...shock tactics..."* to teach. He smiled, saying, *"I did not initially understand your style. You have a strong case. You must write a paper about teaching with pictures!"*

The response to Pictures in AIDucation by the public has been of two extremes, especially in the late 1980s and early 1990s of the epidemic. I have included the experiences and responses between 1989 to 1992 when the Livingstone team and Athlone team were teaching with the popular set of Uganda posters on HIV infection and AIDS. I will start with some negative outcomes or responses:

69

1. Negative outcomes or responses to AIDucation

- Health Programme managers' *"...fear of the unknown"* to endorse Pictures in AIDucation as a cost effective, simple, user-friendly intervention strategy for raising HIV infection and AIDS awareness in the community. Reasons given included; *"...radical...controversial...no one else uses it...shock tactics do not work...behaviour change communication is not only about information...some of the pictures are obscene...some of the images are offensive...we must ask foreign consultants (United Kingdom or America)!"*

- Consultants from "reputable" International Organisations advised government(s) against the use of Pictures in AIDucation as it was *"...too ambitious...radical strategy...studies have shown that scare tactics do not work...images are only for doctors and nurses...shock tactics are old strategies...the public will not understand the messages and might interpret the images wrongly...easy to back-fire with grave consequences...no donor funds for such a programme...we must follow donor criteria!"*

- Elderly traditionalists and gatekeepers of culture walked out of the AIDucation workshops in protest as they felt *"...insulted...were not shown respect...decay of culture...it was un-African...the vagina and penis are not supposed to be shown in public...very rude...these foreigners (Dr Mapara) do not understand our (Botswana) culture...decent traditional way of life is not respected...pornography...a taboo!"*

- One elderly woman stripped naked, into her birthday suit, to show me her *"private parts"* in front of other women as she said, *"...you are going around showing vaginas to everybody!"* I was not showing everybody, I was showing some people. Judgement told me that *"silence was golden"* while the woman was in her birthday suit. That was going to be a wrong place and time to correct her statement. The naked situation warranted silence and eyes looking down, to the floor. The woman's reaction was an extreme reaction, which is not uncommon in many African cultures or countries, where a woman who has felt very insulted, offended, belittled or humiliated "genitally" would take off all her clothes to picture a statement.

- Parents did not want their children to see these pictures as, *"...the pictures will corrupt their morals and innocent young minds...too young for adult things...will contaminate innocent children from decent homes... will lead them to wanting to experiment with sex!"*

- The early church and faith communities would not listen initially, as they were judgemental and had a moralistic view that *"...HIV infection and AIDS are for sinners...for people with loose morals...for people sleeping around and leading promiscuous lives...for people living unbiblical lives...for people who were breaking the commandments in the Bible...for people who are doing wrong things and only reaping what they had sown...for pagans...for non-believers...for infidels...for prostitutes!"*

- Healthcare workers, locally, nationally and internationally were opposed to AIDucation and branded the intervention strategy *"...Shock tactics do not work...what can come from a small district hospital...what research have they (Athlone Hospital) published?"*

- Lack of financial support in the early days from the government authorities because of *"...the radical approach ... not following national guidelines...no money for such programmes!"*

Despite the lack of support, Athlone Hospital persisted on this lonely, picturistic, rough but right path. Athlone Hospital was very lucky that it had a very understanding, down to earth Hospital Advisory Committee that was composed of senior citizens of Lobatse. Athlone Hospital turned to the Hospital Advisory Committee for support. The Committee supported Athlone AIDS Awareness Project financially from its birth to its maturation, until it became a national programme.

2. Positive outcomes or responses to AIDucation

In both Zambia and Botswana, the positive responses were almost the same. Some outcomes were:

- Knowledge base increased at all levels in the local community leading to:
  - Rise in voluntary counselling and testing (VCT) requests before marriage, before pregnancy and in new relationships
  - Increased voluntary counselling and testing to *"Know your status"*
  - Increased early health seeking behaviour as a result of the *"diseases...conditions ...infections"* seen in the clinical pictures
  - Increased *"self-diagnosis"* in some cases, especially for tuberculosis (TB) which has a cure. Athlone had one of the best TB programmes in the country. The secret was that it was a combined TB, HIV infection and AIDS programme from the first day, in 1990. Athlone Hospital was dealing with the *"twin infections"* of TB and HIV infection. Athlone Hospital used both TB and HIV infection to raise awareness of the other infection. TB and HIV are related in more than eighty percent of cases in Africa.

- Controversial cultural practices that were spreading HIV infection were being questioned critically, especially those involving sexual rituals. I recall, while in Livingstone the way I had to beg for a ten minutes slot for Livingstone Anti-AIDS Project to give a talk on HIV infection and AIDS at the 1990 United National Independence Party (UNIP) Convention held in Namwala, Southern Province of Zambia. This would be the equivalent of the annual Labour Party Convention being held in Brighton, United Kingdom. The Livingstone team was given ten minutes, reluctantly, in the main political party's programme for the day. Ten minutes ended up into an hour on the day of the talk, as the politicians engaged in an AIDucated dialogue with the Livingstone Project team, through questions and answers after having given them a talk with the early 1990's Uganda set of posters and pictures. This social intercourse with the politicians was to later play a major role in the stopping of the controversial *"sexual cleansing ritual"* conducted after the death of a spouse in the southern province of Zambia. *"Seeing is believing!"* The politicians saw, believed and acted. *"Seeing is very different from being told."*

- Sexual intercourse, sexuality, will-writing, death and dying became subjects for discussions in AIDucation workshops.

- Increased referral of patients from traditional doctors to health facilities. For Athlone Hospital, the traditional doctors were part of the solution and not part of the problem.

- Formation of support groups for people living with HIV infection and AIDS.

- Training of *"Positive Speakers"* as Livingstone and Athlone Hospitals advocated for *"Greater Involvement of People living with HIV infection and AIDS (GIPA)."*

- Formation of burial societies. Athlone Hospital Burial Society was one of the first in the government hospitals. Coordinated successfully by the Industrial Class.

- Visit to Athlone Hospital by local, national and international AIDS officials from all the continents. One very prominent visitor was General Jerry Rawlings, former President of Ghana, in April 2001. Others included: A *"Why Wait"* delegation from Malawi, TASO officials from Uganda, officials from Zambia National AIDS Council, a positive female speaker from Namibia, a positive speaker from South Africa, World Health Organisation officials, The Red Crescent officials from Geneva, United Nations Development Programme officials, a Brazilian delegation, Bristol Myers Squibb staff, Harvard University scholars, Baltimore University and Family Health International officials.

- Then there was the *"Day of the Journalists"* in 2001 when Athlone Hospital Resource Centre hosted sixteen journalists from Spain, Belgium, Italy, Canada, France and South Africa. The Athlone team which was always very confident "froze" for the first thirty minutes on that day. I was the spokesman, until the team realised that these journalists with all their intimidating cameras and note-pads were just like any other human beings, asking the same questions asked by all other visitors to Athlone Health Resource Centre. After the visitors had gone I asked the Athlone team what had happened to the confident national Athlone AIDS Awareness Project Team. The team had felt a little bit intimidated with the presence of all those white faces, as stated by one of the nurses, *"Ngaka, the resource centre has not seen so many makgoa (white people) in a single day!"*

- Formation and support of community and home based care programmes.

- Improved management of HIV related illnesses including TB, Kaposi's sarcoma and herpes zoster at Athlone Hospital, with locally designed protocols. We had people travelling to Livingstone Hospital in Zambia and Athlone Hospital in Botswana, from hundreds of kilometres away for *"...treatment for AIDS"* – which Livingstone and Lobatse did not have.

- Requests and invitations to facilitate at national workshops increased, including requests from the faith communities, teaching bodies, learning institutions, trade unions and various employing bodies including the Directorate of Public Service Management (DPSM) and Teacher Services Management (TSM). Athlone Hospital would even be reminded by the folks inviting the team, *"...not to forget to come with the pictures."*

- More people, young and old, recommending that Pictures in AIDucation be used in Sex Education in the schools, churches and workplaces in Africa and even in Europe.

Two significant responses at national level

1) Traditional doctors' response

In early 1990s a man with extensive, progressive Kaposi's sarcoma and with severe swellings "elephantiasis" of both legs escaped amputation of both legs because the wife had refused to sign the consent form. Reason given was that Dr Mapara had said in one AIDucation workshop that the condition could be *"...treated with strong drugs."*

The wife to the patient refused to grant permission to the doctors to amputate or cut off both legs so as to stop the Kaposi's sarcoma from spreading. She recalled me saying in one of the AIDucation workshops in the village community hall on discussing pictures of Kaposi's sarcoma that, *"...This (picture of Kaposi's sarcoma of the legs) is not witchcraft or a curse. It is a cancer and it can be treated if brought in early to the hospital."* To cut a long story short, the patient had Kaposi's sarcoma and his blood on HIV testing was found to be HIV negative, which was very significant. The patient was referred to a neighbouring country for a specialist doctor to see him.

The patient was put on very strong drugs for treating Kaposi's sarcoma. His response to the treatment was as expected, the swelling of the legs reduced to almost normal sized legs and feet.

73

Pictures in AIDucation saved the man's legs. The man has both his legs and puts on shoe size number eight. The man literally told and still tells the community of Lobatse that he *"...walks on Edwin's legs!"* The power of observation by a simple woman in the village, who had faith in Pictures in AIDucation, saved her husband's legs. *Seeing is very different from being told.*

The story does not end there. Traditional doctors across the country, who had tried *"traditional treatment"* on the patient, came to hear of this *"...incredible cure"* of an incurable disease. Some went over to see him for themselves, to see *"...the miracle by the small Zambian AIDS' doctor at Athlone Hospital."* Word went round that Dr Mapara must also be *"...a traditional doctor with an added white man's western medical training."* A few of them came to enquire on what medicine had been used to treat the *"witchcraft"*. Athlone Hospital took the opportunity to make arrangements for a session with some of the traditional doctors.

2) "AIDucation-National Tour of Hope"

The climax of Pictures in AIDucation was the Botswana eight weeks *"National Tour of Hope"* from June to July 1997. The Permanent Secretary of The Ministry of Health appointed Athlone Hospital's AIDucation team to travel to the three referral hospitals and six district hospitals to *"...help establish similar programmes like yours (Athlone AIDS Awareness Programme)."*

The long awaited recognition of the *"...controversial...radical...too ambitious...not serious...dreamers...shock tactics...alarmist"* Athlone Hospital AIDS awareness Programme had come of age. The Lobatse project was finally going national. The approach was working and remained robust. The Athlone Hospital Team was sponsored by the government of Botswana on a national assignment, six years after its formation. Athlone Hospital celebrated. It was like Athlone Hospital had won the world cup in football. The *"radical"* Athlone Hospital Team was now being treated as *"National HIV infection and AIDS Consultants"* on a government ticket, with a government BX minibus and a government driver at its disposal. The delegation leader was one of the senior matrons, Mmapula Sechele, from Princess Marina Hospital, the major referral hospital in Gaborone, the capital city of Botswana.

Doors that were tightly shut before were now being opened very wide for the Athlone Hospital Team to enter. The team stayed in the best hotels in the various towns, as Athlone Hospital AIDS Awareness team did what it did best, picturing HIV infection and AIDS. Another 1990 prediction came to pass, that Athlone AIDS Awareness Project would be a national programme before the year 2000, which was also echoed by Noerine Kaleeba in her June 1995 visit to Botswana. The team did not have to say, *"We told you so in 1990!"* The local, village initiated, radical, stubborn, Athlone Hospital AIDS Awareness Project had become one of Botswana's leading National AIDS Programmes, period. The "*local project*" was transformed into a "*national programme.*"

By September 1996 the Vancouver International Conference on AIDS and Sexually Transmitted Infections had announced Botswana's unenviable HIV infection and AIDS prevalence status of being "*...number one*" in the world, having surpassed Uganda and Zambia. Sadly, this is one of the predictions that Athlone Hospital had made in 1990, looking at the early HIV infection and AIDS trend(s) in Botswana and the luke-warm, uncoordinated response. It came to pass, just like many other predictions did.

The Athlone team had earned its "*Consultant status*" in Botswana. The Athlone team was on the road for almost eight weeks, during the national tour, spending three days at each government health facility, not only talking about, but actively picturing HIV infection and AIDS. The health facilities included:

a) Referral hospitals: Lobatse Mental Hospital, Princess Marina Hospital (Gaborone) and Nyangabgwe Hospital (Francistown)

b) District hospitals: Scottish Livingstone Memorial Hospital (Molepolole) Sekgoma Memorial Hospital (Serowe), Selibe-Phikwe Hospital, Palapye Hospital, Mahalapye Hospital and Maun General Hospital.

The Botswana map below shows where the Athlone team travelled to as they pictured HIV infection and AIDS. The team travelled from the South East District to Southern District, Kweneng District, Central District, North East District and finally to Maun in Ngamiland District. The AIDucation pictures have been to those rural and urban places. Athlone covered more than 2 400 kilometres picturing HIV infection and AIDS across the country in 1997. The tour took the Athlone team from Lobatse to Maun and back to Lobatse.

At each hospital visited, the observations by the Athlone Hospital team were depressing and very worrying. Athlone Hospital had no hospital to compare with in Botswana in terms of AIDucation. "*...Athlone Hospital is in a league of its own,*" as stated by many AIDucation participants or visitors to Athlone Hospital. The international visitors to Athlone Hospital helped the team to up their programme by a notch every time they visited.

Similarly, the serious recommendations by the healthcare workers at the hospitals being visited were almost the same and all asked why the "*National Tour of Hope*" had not taken place much earlier in the HIV infection and AIDS epidemics. That was a very difficult question to answer.

MAP OF BOTSWANA – "ATHLONE NATIONAL TOUR OF HOPE"

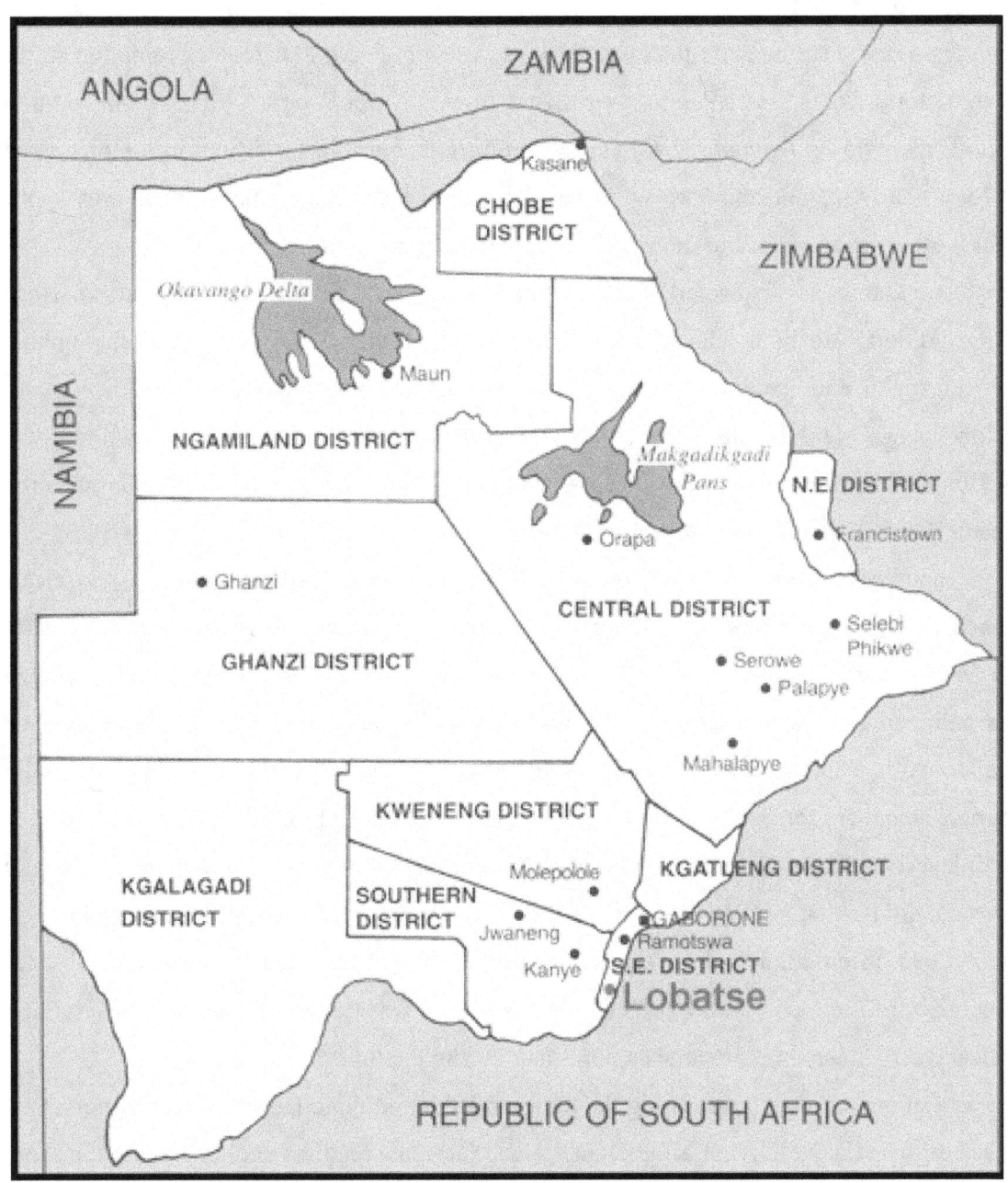

Many doctors and nurses at primary hospitals complained bitterly about being left out of the Athlone Hospital's *"National Tour of Hope"* as the team passed through their villages or towns. The Athlone team could only refer them to headquarters to air their grievances. It was fantastic to be given *"red carpet"* recognition and put in the lime-light after being in the background over the years. It was a dream come true for the*"...full of themselves...arrogant"* Athlone Hospital team.

The tour was a hectic humanitarian mission, conducted by natives of the land. It was soothing that a local village project had become a national programme. It was no mean achievement. The early 1990s' *"stumbling block"* had become the late 1990s' *"stepping stone!"* It was a promotion, from *"...villains"* to victors, from *"...dreamers"* to realists, from *"...shock tactics"* to *"...reality"* and from *"...too ambitious"* to *"...National HIV infection and AIDS consultants."* This was a momentous achievement for a small village team. It was a joyful, wonderful feeling and achievement, only spoilt by the fact that it came seven years and thousands of new infections too late.

The Athlone team was vindicated. The Lobatse community, the Athlone Hospital Advisory Committee, the Athlone Hospital Management Team and healthcare workers were champions. History had been made and that must not be forgotten. Athlone Hospital had laid down many foundations for Botswana's HIV infection and AIDS programmes over the years, including the Botswana National Antiretroviral Therapy Programme. The Lobatse community members are the unsung heroes in Botswana's AIDS control programmes.

That is another reason for this book, **PICTURES IN AIDUCATION - African Communities Talking Sex, AIDS and Pictures**, lest we forget, to document Lobatse's HIV infection and AIDS programmes so as to inspire and motivate other communities out there to believe in themselves and their abundant village or town resources. Village folks only need the confidence and self belief to work wonders. The self-belief is missing in many Africans, including the public health programme managers across the continent and the political leadership.

The Athlone Hospital AIDucation *"National Tour of Hope"* tour was an eye-opener. Many health facilities did not have any HIV infection and AIDS prevention, care and support programme in place. The knowledge, information and resources were very limited. Many healthcare workers did not have comprehensive information on HIV infection and AIDS. It was due to this fact and observation that the team leader, Dr Mapara became the camera-man during the tour.

Dr Mapara stopped giving talks during the tour and let the Athlone Hospital team of nurses do the job, which they did very well. After all, they had given the same lectures and talks, with the same pictures, over five years, since 1992. The rehearsals were over, the curtains were up – it was now show time. Capacity-building and empowerment had taken place over the years. I became a camera man in the background and did more touring and sight-seeing than teaching. I had a capable team, in the *"...A-Team"*, as Athlone Hospital AIDS Awareness team was often called.

After the national tour, the Athlone team conducted a post-mortem which was quick, precise and conclusive. In summary, Botswana had a pending national disaster of unfolding proportions coming. It was from the *"National Tour of Hope"* that the recommendation and the idea of the Athlone Hospital Health Resource Centre was conceived. It was not an American or Zambian idea. It was a Botswana idea. The plan or initiative was for Athlone Hospital to become a *"Public Health School of Pictures in AIDucation"* for training healthcare workers from the other government and non-governmental organisations, schools, churches, faith communities, workplaces and other community based organisations. Athlone Hospital had the *"...niche"* or strength of Pictures in AIDucation, as an awareness raising intervention strategy, which no other organisation had in Botswana. *"Seeing is believing"* and *"Seeing is very different from being told!"*

The dream was for Athlone Hospital AIDS awareness Programme to become what Chikankata Salvation Army Hospital AIDS Programme was to Zambia or The AIDS Support Organisation (TASO) to Uganda or Terrence Higgins Trust (THT) to United Kingdom. If you are an AIDS activist and you do not know about these international programmes, make sure that you do your home-work before you go to Africa as a Consultant, invited by the African governments.

Athlone Hospital working with the other Lobatse stake-holders of the District multi-sectoral AIDS Committee (DMSAC) and armed with the first hand findings, from the *"National Tour of Hope"*, wrote up a project proposal for the development of The Athlone Health Resource Centre and handed it to the authorities for approval and funding. Unfortunately, the proposal for the first Health Resource Centre in Botswana was thrown into the dust-bin by the authorities in 1998, as the familiar words came back, *"...too ambitious...duplication of programmes...not done before...no money...budget too big...special donor fund criteria...will consult foreign consultants!"* History was repeating itself and Athlone Hospital did not have the time to waste or to wait. Athlone Hospital had waited seven years to be heard. Every day was precious. Every day meant hundreds of preventable infections missed. Every day meant hundreds of new AIDS patients to bury in the near future.

There is an African saying that talks of three types of people in the world:

1. Those people who want to make things happen
2. Those people who make things happen
3. Those people who wonder what happened.

People who make things happen

The Athlone family belonged to the group of people who made things happen. The Athlone team approached the Hospital Advisory Committee and took the *"Athlone Way"* again, that had given birth to the Athlone AIDS Awareness Programme in 1990. The Athlone team believed that the Lobatse community would come to its rescue again. The Lobatse community did not disappoint Athlone Hospital. The *"seed money"* was given to the hospital, by the Lobatse community through the successful businessman and Hospital Advisory Committee Patron Mr Asmal Goolam (MHSRIP). The seed germinated and the first Health Resource Centre in Botswana was born at Athlone Hospital on 30th November 1999. The centre was officially opened by the late Patron, Mr Asmal Goolam.

It is important to note and emphasise that the money was raised from the community members of Lobatse. The Ministry of Health and the National AIDS Coordinating Agency (NACA) had not given Athlone Hospital any funding for setting up the Athlone Health Resource Centre. The foundation was laid by the people of Lobatse, who had faith in the potential of their district hospital, Athlone Hospital. They dug deep in their pockets, for their health and well being.

After one year of the Athlone Health Resource Centre rendering services to the community, the long expected good news was delivered through the national press, on 6th December 2000. The local media documented the headline news, which you can read on the web or the internet that,

"Athlone Resource Centre is Number One!"

(Source: Botswana Press Agency (2000 December 6) *Athlone Resource Centre is Number One*. Daily News Online, Available:http://www.gov.bw /cgi-bin/news.cgi?d20001206. Accessed 7 October 2004)

Responses to AIDucation at international level

While based in the borough of Brent in London, England and working for Community Health Action Trust (CHAT), formerly Brent and Harrow Community Health Projects (BHCHP), we have continued with Pictures in AIDucation, since 2003, in the local and national workshops.

It is a "deja vu" of Livingstone and Lobatse. I am going through the same steps of resistance to change, bargaining and reluctant acceptance. The AIDucation workshops have taken me to various towns and audiences in London. I have travelled out of London to Birmingham, Cambridge, Leicester, Norwich, Oxford, Reading, Sheffield, Stafford and Yorkshire picturing HIV infection and AIDS. The AIDucation sessions are similar to the *"National Tour of Hope"* in Botswana, of 1997. History is repeating itself. It is just a matter of time.

Every time I am invited out of London to present on AIDucation, I relieve the *"National Tour of Hope"* in Botswana. I can see Mma Sechele (Matron – Princess Marina Hospital), Boile Kgaodi, Mma Mokganedi, Dorothy Keokgale (Athlone Hospital "A Team") and Kenneth the driver from Princess Marina Hospital. I re-live and travel that journey or tour every year since 1997.

History is repeating itself in England. After a year of Community Health Action Trust's (CHAT) Community Resource Centre operating, it has been recognised and documented by the powers that be as a *"best practice"* or *"...option 2"* community based voluntary counselling and testing centre.

England's HIV infection and AIDS organisations trying to set up community based voluntary counselling and testing centres (VCT) are advised to set up the community based VCT the CHAT way ("Option 2") or originally the Athlone Hospital way, of Lobatse in Botswana. The North learns from the South.

Comments on AIDucation in England

At the end of the AIDucation sessions in London, I usually send the participants an electronic version of the AIDucation evaluation form for comments. Here are some of the comments received and documented in Table 1-HeC, from United Kingdom. The European comments are almost like in Africa, with almost the same standard recommendations.

In Africa, after all the AIDucation workshops we had an evaluation form that we handed out to the participants to fill in. We asked the participants to write down their comments, both positive and negative that would help Athlone Hospital improve on the future AIDucation sessions. In every single workshop, since 1992, there had been comments and suggestions to make Pictures in AIDucation a national intervention strategy. The Athlone Team had religiously reported these unedited recommendations to the relevant authorities.

The paradox of the comments was and still is that the lay community members or grassroots folks living with HIV infection and AIDS everyday, want Pictures in AIDucation to be used as a teaching style, while the doctors, scientists and researchers, usually in the air-conditioned offices saw contrary and call it, *"Shock tactics do not work!"*

There are still several people who cannot *"...see AIDS..."* or relate with AIDS, as AIDS is invisible, even in Europe. Erroneously, in some western countries HIV infections and AIDS are depicted as *"...diseases for gay people, Africans and intravenous drug users."* That implies that if one is not from the gay community or African community or intravenous drug user community then they are safe from HIV infection or AIDS. How sad that people can think that way in this age and era of massive information on HIV infection and AIDS.

Sadly many people realise it and see AIDS too late, when it is now visible in the family, the home, the school, the church or the work place. "Pictures in AIDucation" is for the *"picturate"* community while HIV infection and AIDS literature is usually for the literate community. Whereas

Pictures in AIDucation can be for both the literate and the picturate we cannot say the same for HIV infection and AIDS literature, which is only for the literate. One does not need rocket science to appreciate this very basic fact about effective communication.

It is a known fact that people remember 80% of what they see as compared to 20% of what they hear. So why not picture HIV infection and AIDS? There have been hundreds of comments about AIDucation. These comments have come through workshops, seminars and online discussions. Of the comments, 98% of the comments have been positive and advocate for Pictures in AIDucation, while 2% have been negative, sceptical and would definitely want more information.

Furthermore some comments came from online discussions held between 5th February 2007 and 22nd February 2007, where I was a co-moderator in an online discussion on the same topic of *"Pictures in AIDucation."* The online discussion was hosted by Health e Communication and Communication Initiative.

Some of the comments are from people who read the articles:

- PLOS Medicine article of December 2004, volume 1, issue 3 entitled *"Picturing AIDS: Using Images to raise Community Awareness"*.

- SAFAIDS News 3 September 2003 article: *"Opinion – Pictures as a Health Promotion Strategy in Addressing HIV Infection and AIDS in Developing Countries"*.

- Some of the comments on AIDucation are from people who read the Communication Initiative Strategic Thinking article *"Picturing AIDS: Using Images to Raise Community Awareness."* A number of the comments are from the AIDucation workshop participants, who have been documented on the Communication Initiative website:

http://www.comminit.com/healthecomm/top-tens.php?showdetails=188

The Slides are very informative. Seeing is believing [Western Europe]

Illustrates importance of organizations such as TALC. [Global]

Very useful material, keep it up. [Western Europe]

I found the information very useful indeed and thanks so much for forwarding it [East & Southern Africa]

I also agree that the pictures are a very useful health communication material especially in developing country. Would you please send me a soft/hard copy or the TALC educational slide sets?

I find this material to be very useful and hope that it can be more widely made available. [East & Southern Africa]

Thanks for the good work, greetings from Total Community Mobilisation (TCM) [East & Southern Africa]

I am currently developing health promotion programme for Black and Ethnic Minority Community in Surrey, predominantly white community and I believe these resources would be mostly useful in reaching this targeted community as you have rightly put it we believe in seeing. [Western Europe]

I wish I saw the pictures five years ago. I would have supported my brother better. He had that herpes zoster rash two times. We did not know what it was. We thought it was skin cancer. The pictures must be shown to all school children as they are sexually very active, careless and with many pregnancies and sex diseases like chlamydia. Pictures are good for us to see what the nurses and doctors tell us about AIDS. [Western Europe]

The programme gives a true image of what sexual health is about and sensitises the general public about the intensity of the havoc caused by sexually transmitted infections. The use of pictures in educations has had a definite positive impact on the participants of my sexual health training sessions. It is definitely working. [Western Europe]

I used to find pictures of AIDS patients repugnant too, but now I realise it is worth giving the picture education a try in future presentations. I hope such pictures do not dampen people's libido altogether. Now that the African population has been essentially decimated by AIDS, we need to procreate more. How do we Africans deal with this conundrum? [West Africa]

I believe using pictures as a means of teaching is very useful and communicate well to your audience. [Western Europe]

That pictures & slides really help in getting the message across. [Global]

Dear Sir, I studied the glimpses of your article very thoroughly and found a topic for my research. I have decided to use this idea in the context of Pakistan that how pictures could affect peoples' behaviour in averting them from the risk of AIDS. [South Asia]

This method is very educative and straight- forward. Sometimes language can be a barrier to effective communication hence the use of pictures is imperative. However, some pictures could have a negative impact on people living with HIV when dealing with secondary prevention. Nevertheless this method is easily monitored and evaluated to facilitate the measuring of the long term impact. Well done Edwin no wonder you are so popular at HAAZ support group in London and the local community in Brent and Harrow. [Western Europe]

This is a simple but most effective way of imparting knowledge and creating an unforgettable impact on an audience. [East & Southern Africa]

I have had the pleasure of working with Dr. Mapara and I look forward to further opportunities to learn from his knowledge and expertise in this field. [Global]

"A picture is worth a thousand words". These pictures make our work as health educators much easier, especially as a resource that we can access so readily, I believe that health educators can access them from anywhere in the world. Find more materials so that over time, the picture bank becomes bigger and bigger. Keep the spirit of sharing these invaluable resources. Best regards. [East & Southern Africa]

I strongly believe Dr Mapara is right in using pictures to educate on AIDS. Having seen the pictures myself, I still have that imprinted in my memory and feel once I saw the pictures, I truly believed. There are so many myths and stories that surround AIDS and the pictures tell only one story: You will contract AIDS if you do not protect yourself against it. AIDS has been looked at as an "African problem" but that is not the case. With the financial migration of Africans and Asians to Europe and America, political asylum seekers and refugees, this is something that the entire world should be worried about and continue to do something about. Pictures are just one way of trying to combat AIDS as there are several other ways. I congratulate Dr Mapara and urge him to continue. [East & Southern Africa]

This is simply fantastic. Keep up the good work. [East & Southern Africa]

This resource deserves additional rating. The resource is not just fantastic, but it is indeed what the world needs as indeed what Dr. Mapara says, *"seeing is believing"*. The resource can be used in every situation, i.e. teaching, HIV campaigns and even in hospitals. I propose the resource be adopted by World Health Organisation (WHO). Saying more would spoil the soup. Congratulations and keep up the good work. [East & Southern Africa]

The resource is informative and up to date making suitable reading for the work we do. [Western Europe]

Thank you for offering me the opportunity to read your article in SAFAIDS and also for your reference to TALC UK materials. I was quite fascinated by your approach which is appropriate as individuals may not have a concept (mental picture) of what is HIV and how it could be developed into full blown AIDS. I suppose the initial reaction of the community may be that of denial, but in the end, through perseverance and the belief in your ideas have won the minds and demonstrated the importance of knowledge over ignorance. The multifaceted nature of the condition is clearly depicted in the SAFAIDS news. [Western Europe]

Very useful material, physical evidence of what is heard [East & Southern Africa].

This material is very useful. I was wondering if this or some of the material could be translated to be used by the community health workers in the grassroots. And educating through pictures is useful in that pictures do not need many words to get the message through. [East & Southern Africa]

The Resource is valuable - it should be transmitted to ZANARA and the National Aids Council in Zambia for distribution in Public work places in order to increase awareness and knowledge among public workers. TALC in particular should intensely sensitise and shock most persons - this action could bring reality in the minds of most that under estimate the impact and consequences of AIDS [East & Southern Africa]

Thanks for sending me this resource, it made very interesting reading and will help me in my studies in Health Promotion. Please, always keep me posted in any Health Promotion materials. [West Africa]

I have been involved in the war against HIV infection and AIDS since 1991. The slides are quite helpful. People in this part of the world where I live believe in seeing than just hearing [West Africa]

Being a minister of religion I learnt a lot when I attended the WORD conference in Norwich and I believe using such material to teach young people will be a good idea in the church community. I can recommend for the materials to be used mostly in Africa where I think the problem is paramount. May the Lord be with you as you work hard to save the entire world. We welcome you in Tanzania. [East & Southern Africa]

Excellent [Global].

In my culture *"...seeing is believing".* We are also working with people who may not academically understand the medical terms so a picture will be self explanatory. They can even use a picture in association with a condition they have seen in friends, family etc. Pictures alone are not the best but it should go with information that will help people to make the right choices [East & Southern Africa]

I attended the use of pictorial materials as media of information and awareness on HIV / AIDS at a Workshop in Monks Park Primary Care Clinic in September 2006. It was unique and proved to be an effective way of providing information to audience of both the developing and developed countries and to the Africans in particular. This technique should be adopted as a modern way for global education and knowledge on this global plague. [Global]

AIDucation has received 50 positive comments from readers, to date. We must re-visit health promotion and include pictures in our talks. [East & Southern Africa]

EDITOR"S NOTE: These comments come from the author of this article.
Five years in the UK has shown me that UK needs this intervention strategy. It is just a matter of time, before the AIDucation strategy is used. Hope it will not be too late by then. People do not know about HIV infection and AIDS. They want to "see" HIV infection and AIDS. The resource evaluates a strategy being used in the borough of Brent to teach and share experiences in raising HIV infection and AIDS awareness through pictures. The 50 Health e Communication comments and ratings are making a statement. Should the

Health Promotion curriculum be revised? [Global]

In India HIV infection and AIDS is spreading fast from high risk groups to common people posing a great threat. Using "Pictures" is a good idea amongst the less educated people. It has worked in some African countries, and should be helpful in spreading better awareness about HIV / AIDS and in bringing about the desired behavioural change. [South Asia]

Very good and should continue [Western Europe]

I think working with pictures is great. However, this should not be restricted to developing countries alone as it is always assumed that people living in highly developed countries are very aware of these issues. This assumption contributes to the rising sexually transmitted infections (STI) infections in young people in some of these countries. Let us not just talk about them. Let us see what we are talking about too! [Western Europe]

This is great Edwin. Keep it up. I am sure in the new year, God willing, we shall surely see more. Apologies for the delay in responding but I was indisposed. [East & Southern Africa]

In my wider experience of Development Education we have found that what people see has a lasting impact on them then when one talks at them. So there is a definite place for pictures in AIDS Education [East & Southern Africa]

I have had the privilege of attending seminars and workshops on Dr Mapara's Pictures in AIDucation. I have used them in my practice as trainee social worker and intend to continue doing so. Based on Mapara's workshops, I have passed on information to friends, relatives and people that I work with. My focus is now targeted at my university which has a very large population of students. Pictures tell you more and I have never forgotten the pictures I saw 3 years ago when I first attended Dr Mapara's workshop. I hope more people will use pictures to tell a story and emphasise the need for us to work in collaboration in relation to HIV infection and AIDS. I wish Mapara continued success in this fight against AIDS. [Global]

Would like to see a link to the tools (pictures) that he utilizes so I can better understand and assess for myself. [North America]

Whilst I don't agree like all the pictures, I do believe that their use is very effective to some people [Western Europe]

Do you recommend using this resource in the UK? I would have loved to use it in churches in Kent [Western Europe]

I personally, even from my place of work, we use HIV infection and AIDS pictures to reach out to the community because after discussions then you wrap up with real pictures you find that you get powerful response especially people accessing counselling and testing. I think if all organisations dealing in HIV infection and AIDS can use clinical picture people will take things seriously because they are seeing real people. [East & Southern Africa]

The resource is important in sexual health awareness campaigns with young people. The target group pays more attention to pictures and seem to participate more actively than in other forms of communication. [Western Europe]

This is an effective medium of communication on HIV infection and AIDS. It is relevant, provocative thoughtful. [East & Southern Africa]

Dr Mapara has successfully produced a tool to tackle one of the major barriers to health promotion and health education - getting the message across to a wide and culturally diverse population. I am particularly impressed with his engagement of young people around HIV infection and AIDS and sexual health generally. His passion and commitment to this approach captivate audiences which must ultimately lead to community involvement and action. [Western Europe]

Using pictures in educating people is very important especially for communities where English is not their first language or have low levels of education. More so "seeing is believing" and it can make a bigger impact. I have had the opportunity to use this material in some of our trainings and our users found it very beneficial. Continue the good work. [Western Europe]

Is there an organisation that could share some of their resources with us? (graphic images) [East & Southern Africa]

I am a Social worker, Pastor and Sexual Health Promotion Specialist, with 22 years of experience. I am a founder of Widows and Orphans Relief and Development Trust (WORD). As a pastor I have seen negative attitudes towards people living with HIV and a blame culture of immorality so rife coupled with ignorance as the church has closed its ears to the information. I have taken it as a challenge for our organisation to work with the church in Africa to make them take on HIV as part of their agenda. The use of pictures will just be the quickest way of making them understand. As Edwin says "seeing is believing." As a sexual health promotion specialist we have worked with Edwin during our different promotion days such as World AIDS Day and others. We have also used them in training with primary care staff. There are a very useful tool and will not hesitate to refer others to them. [Western Europe]

Using pictures in education for HIV infection and AIDS presents the reality of HIV infection and not the imaginary which in most cases does not give the right image. AIDucation is instrumental for primary prevention and as an education tool for health providers. [Western Europe]

I will be grateful to learn more about HIV information messages to improve on Prevention.[East & Southern Africa]

We use the pictures for our seminars and work shops, although take some precautions for the elderly [Western Europe]

Most adults remember what they see more than what they hear. So the use of pictures as a strategy in AIDS Education and Prevention work is an excellent one [East & Southern Africa]

This is a very useful resource that need to be replicated in our communities in Kenya. [East & Southern Africa]

Having watched the slides during my visit to the U.K in the year that just ended, I strongly believe they are the best way to reach even the illiterate masses of many developing countries and also the already developed countries and I am also A BELIEVER OF SEEING IS BELIEVING as the saying goes. How I wish Malawi which has been one of the hardest hit in the sub-Sahara was considered, and accorded an opportunity to benefit greatly from Dr Mapara. How I wish he was here yesterday than the unknown tomorrow. [Western Europe]

Useful picture to be used to educate people, people need to understand these things by visualizing. [East & Southern Africa]

The pictures does wonders [East & Southern Africa]

Very interesting and useful site, I would like to continue with it .Thanks. [Latin America]

Simply Excellent!! [Global]

The methods used by Dr Mapara are the most effective that I have ever experienced. They offer a visual impact that is extremely effective. I have seen the impact that these pictures have had on members of the public and I would recommend that every person who values their way of life take the time to investigate this method of health promotion. [East & Southern Africa]

Refreshingly innovative, frank and positive approach. [East & Southern Africa]

Jokes aside, seeing is believing. This is probably the only way some people can be made to believe that there is AIDS. Keep up the good work. [East & Southern Africa]

Useful to acknowledge input from regional examples e.g. TASO-Uganda. This shows the practicality of interventions in almost similar settings. TBA and PMTCT figures, Botswana have some impressive figures!! Article has a genuine applicability on a wider regional scale. [East & Southern Africa]

Hello, I really need such materials (pictures) to use it in my academic field and to do health Education campaigns in South Sudan. [East & Southern Africa]

An educative instrument keep up the good work [Western Europe]

I think pictures or images talk more than we do. For me it is a good way to make people aware the diseases good luck Dr Mapara [West Africa]

As the population in Africa is in majority illiterate the best way to spread such important information is by pictures in the sense that Africans are more visual memory. This method already in use in Ivory Coast has helped a lot to bring the population at an acceptable level of knowledge of this calamity. [West

Africa]

I have found that visual aids / picture are the most effective way to reach young people with the effects of sexually transmitted infections. This is knowledge that I have gained from previous experience, working with young people. Although tutors have sometimes found the images offensive, young people have not, they have seen and acted by way of seeking more advice and resources to practice safe sex. [Western Europe]

Source: Health e Communication, 2007. *Picturing AIDS: Using Images to Raise Community Awareness.* Available: http:/www.comminit.com/healthecomm/top-tens.php?showdetails=188

AIDUCATION

Multi-sectoral approach is needed if we are to stop the spread of HIV infection and AIDS. Governments, schools, faith communities, work places, clubs, non-governmental organisations (NGO) and

Community based organisations (CBO) should all be involved in AIDucation.

Needles and syringes or *"the works"* should not be shared. The same message stands for people who attend "clinics" of traditional doctors. Carry your own razor blade.

8. SHORT COURSES IN AIDUCATION

> *"Smoke does not affect honey-bees alone; honey-gatherers are also affected."*

African saying

Community involvement

A lot of African communities or village members would like to play an active role when it comes to HIV infection and AIDS prevention, care and support initiatives or any other activities. The problem is that they do not know where to start from. They lack the knowledge and simply have no basic HIV infection and AIDS syllabus, guidelines or curriculum to follow or learn from.

The Livingstone and Lobatse programmes had people approaching them in Zambia and Botswana respectively with good intentions but no direction. Requests came in such as:

- *"Can you come and talk to us about the genetics of AIDS?"*
- *" We would like your views on the science of AIDS"*
- *"To discuss the origin of AIDS and if it is true"*
- *"To debate the transmission of AIDS through mosquitoes"*
- *"To confirm that AIDS is not an education strategy against teenage pregnancy."*

The list is endless. We had to work out what exactly the requests were trying to address. In Botswana, Athlone Hospital had made a standard AIDucation programme to help community folks and others seeking assistance. People wanted to be informed, to be taught, to be educated and empowered on sexually transmitted infections including HIV infection and AIDS that had caused such suffering and misery.

HIV infection and AIDS was forever being talked about on the radio. It was therefore not uncommon to hear in whispers and low tone voices that someone died of "*...The radio disease...the four letter word...the disease most talked about these days...the disease of the blankets...the disease of the foreigners...Mapara's disease...Mavunika sign!*"

Athlone Hospital designed a five days course in the hope of preparing the country for what was, sadly, yet to come. The response to HIV infection and AIDS in Botswana, in the early 1990s was like in most African countries, lukewarm. There was initial denial and procrastination. Time was being wasted looking for whom to blame. It was believed that AIDS was *"...a disease of foreigners."* Many locals thought that AIDS was not an issue in Botswana. Sadly it was a very major issue in the hospital wards in Athlone Hospital, in September 1990, the month of my first appointment.

AIDucation is about shared information, education, responsibilities and community engagement. The guidelines have not changed much, since 1992, apart from the addition of the Prevention of Mother to Child Transmission (PMTCT) of HIV infection, Post Exposure Prophylaxis (PEP) and the introduction of Antiretroviral Therapy (ART) or anti-HIV drugs.

The AIDucation guidelines have been used to develop short courses, since 1992 at Athlone Hospital, Botswana to 2008 at Community Health Action Trust (CHAT) in London. Some content;

1. **Sexually transmitted infections**
   o Knowledge about the other sexually transmitted infections is required before talking about HIV infection and AIDS. It cannot be over emphasised.
     ▪ Infections are discussed broadly with the common infections highlighted including syphilis, genital ulcers, chlamydia, candida (thrush), genital warts, gonorrhoea, herpes, buboes, discharges from the penis and vagina.
     ▪ Sexually transmitted infections in babies are discussed to. General sexual health talk is essential before talking about HIV infection and AIDS.
     ▪ Sexual health talks initiated free talks about *"taboo"* subjects, namely sexual intercourse, sexuality, culture and death.

2. **Basic facts of HIV infection and AIDS**
   o Knowledge about the virus - how it causes ill health, why it is different from other viruses, how it is transmitted, the routes of transmission and prevention strategies.
     ▪ Discussed the myths, rumours, stories, traditional beliefs and facts of HIV infection and AIDS.
     ▪ Discussed the ways or routes of HIV infection and the body fluids that are infectious, so as to remove the element of fear in relatives who would finally nurse their patients living with HIV infection and AIDS in the homes.
     ▪ Principles of prevention strategies and universal precautions are discussed. Waste management in hospitals and homes is discussed.

3. **Clinical manifestations or ways of presentation of HIV infection and AIDS**
   o Diseases, infections and conditions discussed included herpes zoster (shingles), Kaposi's sarcoma, swellings of the glands, weight loss, chronic diarrhoea, tuberculosis (TB), chest infections, candida (thrush), skin rashes and AIDS in children.

- Discussed the common diseases seen in people with HIV infections and how they can mimic other diseases or conditions such as tuberculosis (TB), malnutrition, diabetes, alcoholism, cancer or allergic drug reactions.
- Stressed that it was not witchcraft or curses put on families by jealous relatives. Information was shared on how to treat some of these diseases or ailments.
- Emphasised the importance of seeking early medical advice when sick.

4. **Prevention, care and support**
   - Shared information on counselling, home based care, pregnancy and HIV infection, care for orphans, hygiene, sanitation, condom use, social work, intervention strategies and the role of the media.
     - Discussed types of counselling and the role of social workers, role of the media, the relatives, the community members and healthcare workers in HIV infection and AIDS care.
     - Discussed issues of shared confidentiality and shared responsibilities.
     - Shared experiences on home-based care, orphan care and other workable care and support strategies in the real world of living with HIV infection and AIDS. Examples of programmes shared were mostly from Africa – Botswana, South Africa, Uganda, Zambia and Zimbabwe.

AIDUCATION

Orphans and vulnerable children are on the increase world wide. These children are human beings, just like you and me. They need love, care, support, compassion and nurturing.

Prevention of the mother to child transmission of HIV infection programme should be supported. Babies can be born HIV negative despite the mother having HIV infection or being HIV positive.

PART 2

Community stories in AIDucation

- o   Reality of HIV infection and AIDS

  - o   *"Worms in the condoms"*

- o   HIV as a *"chameleon"* or *" bird in motion"*

  - o   *"Changing skin of the virus"*

- o   *"Undetectable levels"* of HIV infection

  - o   *"Betrayal by pastor"*

  - o   *"HIV is too clever"*

  - o   *"Oral what!?"*

  - o   Man's emotions and sex

- o   Talking stigma, discrimination and isolation

- o   PMTCT and *"broadcasting"* HIV results

  - o   Monthly periods or at *"the moon"*

- o   *"Die a little bit more to qualify for AIDS treatment!"*

  - o   *"Test for everything!"*

- o   Rape and post exposure prophylaxis (PEP)

- o   Traditional or home deliveries of babies

  - o   Sex education.

African AIDucation participants

9. PICTURING HIV INFECTION AND AIDS

"A picture is worth a thousand words."

English saying

The Athlone Hospital AIDucation workshops

In this second part of the book, comments and quotations from the various AIDucation workshops have been shared and written down. For the intended learning outcomes on each slide or picture, the author has called it **"African Communities Talking Sex, AIDS and Pictures (ACTSAP)."** These are some of the messages that must come out of that picture during the dialogue or discussion. Ask the participants to always tell you what they see in the pictures. Build the discussions from what the participants say. You will be surprised at what you will learn or unlearn.

The author has gone on to give a few **"TIPS" – Talking information points and stories** – from past AIDucation workshops in Africa. You do not necessarily need to use these TIPS for the discussion to bring out these messages. The TIPS are just to guide you or some loud thoughts.

Effective communication differs with cultures. There are some tribes or cultures that have no problem talking about the penis and vagina. Some will even call a person by these names or organs. Other communities will not use such *"...offensive ...vulgar...insults ...obscene...unspeakable ...rude...too heavy for the tongue..."* vocabulary or language.

With each black and white picture a true community story or two is narrated that took place, hoping to bring out a lesson or two from each. Names, places and dates have been deliberately left out or changed. Most of the talk or *"quotations"* are written the way they were said or spoken, literal translation, with little editing and in some cases sounding like broken English or poor grammar.

For you to appreciate the colour slides and scientific text by Dr Cathy Vaughan and Dr Wendy Holmes, refer to: **HIV Infection – Virology and Transmission (Africa) HIVT-F Slides 1-24 (November 2002).** The modules are available and distributed by TALC, St Albans, England. The TALC website is www.talcuk.org .

In fact, you might have to use these modules written by Dr Cathy Vaughan and Dr Wendy Holmes first, with the initially intended audience or target group of healthcare workers in the hospitals and clinics before getting into those schools, colleges, universities, churches, mosques, traditional institutions, work places, barracks, camps, street corners and social events.

The author received a few bruises to have Pictures in AIDucation accepted as a practical teaching method. It was not all rosy and smooth sailing. Do not be discouraged. Where there is a will there is a picture, sorry, there is a way!

HIVT-F 1: The rapid spread of AIDS

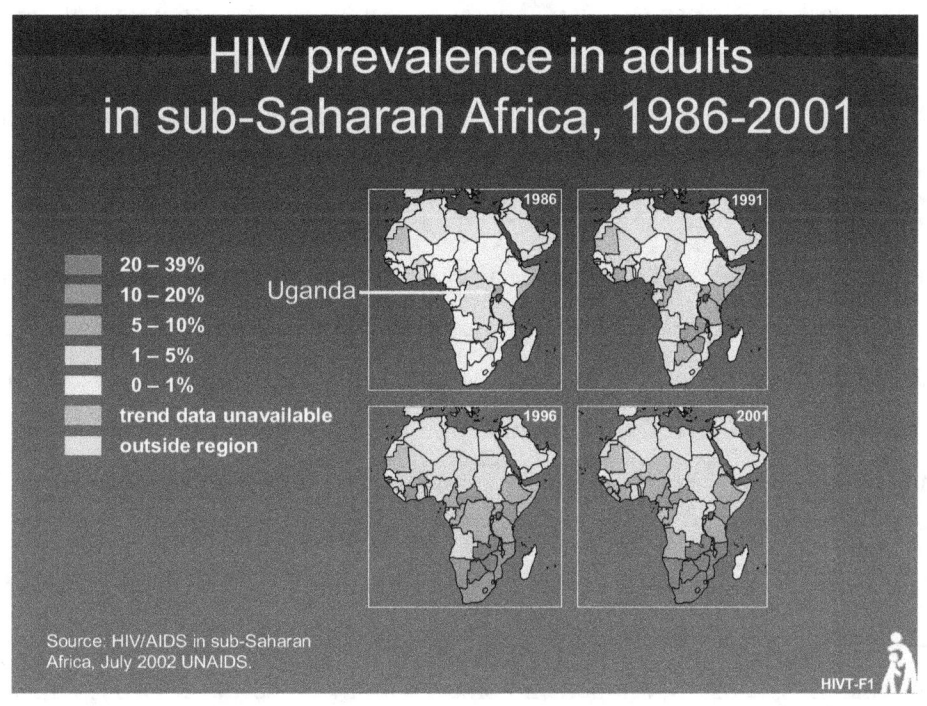

African Communities Talking Sex, AIDS and Pictures (ACTSAP)

- Talk about the world and national (your country) numbers of people living with HIV infection and AIDS

- Talk about sentinel surveillance studies or surveys and how they are conducted or done in your country

- Give a human face to the numbers of people living with HIV infection and AIDS.

Talking information points and stories ("TIPS")

o Start with the global overview and numbers from the latest World Health Organisation, UNAIDS Report, Avert or any other reliable source. Keep it short and simple. Statistics, graphs and numbers can be boring for many of us in the community.

o Discuss sentinel surveillance studies (SSS) and how they are done in your country. Sounds too technical - "jargon"- but not to worry as it is simple and straight forward.

o Explain that the studies are done over a three months period in either pregnant women or mothers, patients with sexually transmitted infections (genital ulcers) and in tuberculosis (TB) patients.

o It is only during these studies that blood is taken and screened or tested for HIV infection without permission, consent or counselling of the client or person being tested. This is called anonymous testing. No names and no addresses. Simply a blood sample with no identity.

o Official permission to conduct the study is given by the Permanent Secretary or Minister of Health, Ministry of Health, working with guidelines from World Health Organisation (WHO).

o Explaining the study brings AIDS into the community, amongst us and it ceases being too academic. The results are about us in the village or town.

o The four pictures of Africa are discussed in depth showing the growth of the epidemic from 1986 to 2001. Use updated recent slides if possible, but do keep the 1986 and 1991 pictures. The red coloured areas on the map are pointed out to show the aggressive, rapid spread of HIV infection and AIDS across the continent.

o Uganda was once the *"AIDS Capital"* but now it is no longer so. Which country is the *"AIDS Capital?"* It is no laughing matter. It is a life and death situation.

o Southern African countries are highly affected, including the "rich" countries of South Africa and Botswana. Is it a disease of poverty? South Africa and Botswana are two of Africa's richest countries, more developed in some areas than the developed countries. Very true. What happened?

Community talks about "...*the reality*" of HIV infection

o Participants appreciated the knowledge shared and some were stunned at the fact of *"...real HIV blood test results...frightening truth of figures"* of the local population.

o Some village folks blamed the government for not telling the people tested about their (anonymous) results and hence *"...spreading the infection (HIV) more in the village!"*

o There were some emotional reactions and comments such as *"... Mapara and his team are killing our people with their tests for statistics and research...He cannot do this with his own people (Zambians)!"*

o Why the rapid spread? Good discussion point.

o Comparisons between northern and southern Africa were often discussed. Quotations picked at random:

- *"Why the differences?"*
- *"Is it to do with sexual, cultural practices in Southern Africa?"*
- *"Does polygamy have a role to play?"*
- *"Africans are not as promiscuous as white people!"*

- *"Do male and female circumcisions have something to do with the spread of HIV infection?"*
- *"Commonwealth countries or countries that were colonised by the British Empire are hard hit compared to the French colonised countries! Why?"*
- *"Christian countries where the Catholics have refused the use of the condoms are affected more!"*
- *"Christianity encourages silence about sexual matters."*
- *Good people...well brought up people do not talk about sex."*
- *AIDS will keep on spreading, as long as the church keeps quiet!"*

This picture can be very *"...politically supercharged"* with participants bringing in their beliefs of where HIV infection and AIDS came from with a lot of conspiracy theories such as *"...the West wants to kill off the Africans...the West manufactured AIDS in the laboratories...germ warfare...condoms are contaminated with AIDS...The Pope and the Vatican do not support condom use because they know the truth!"*

Whatever the origin, that is not important. We have a duty to society, to Africa, to prevent new infections and to support those people living with or have been affected by HIV infection and AIDS. We must reduce stigma and we must speak for people living with HIV infection or living with AIDS in our communities. *"No one chooses to become infected with HIV!"*

This first picture sets the stage or scenario for the next few days, so to say, if discussed frankly and honestly. It is worth nudging, provoking and encouraging the participants to talk their minds and hearts out. There is no silly comment or stupid question in AIDucation. All observations, comments and questions are very valuable.

Community talks about *"...worms in the condom"*

An elderly woman in an AIDucation workshop called me aside during tea-break, *"My son can I ask you a question, that I could not ask you in the hall?"* The old woman looked visibly disturbed. *"Go ahead mum, feel very free and ask,"* I responded. *"Is it true that there are worms in the condoms?"* she asked. *"No, there are no worms in the condoms,"* I answered, truthfully. *"What makes you say that there are worms in the condoms?"* I asked politely. She elaborated as she held her left arm high, as if holding a condom that had been removed from a packet. *"When you hold a condom high against the sun, you can see the worms* (melting lubricant or oil) *coming down by the sides and they (worms) collect at the bottom of the condom* (lubricant or oil).*These worms are HIV that the Americans have put in the condom we are told!"*

She was so clear in her description and no wonder she had to ask for clarification. Can you picture or imagine the condom's sides touching each other and seeming to move as the oil or lubricant melted and collected at the bottom of the condom like semen?

After the workshop, I asked some nurses at Athlone Hospital if they had heard of such an incredible story before. I was shocked when a few nurses said that they had heard of it and they all named the same village that the old lady had mentioned during the AIDucation workshop.

This old woman's question made the Athlone Hospital team travel to the named village where this "story" was circulating to go and dismiss it and explain the truth on condoms and the oil or lubricant in the condom.

There are no *"worms"* or HIV infection or AIDS in the condoms. The Americans have not put in HIV infection or AIDS in the condoms. The Americans do not manufacture all the condoms that Africa uses. The condoms come from all over the world, including China. We once had to send the Chinese condoms back. There was a size problem.

LESSONS LEARNT

- It is important to try to follow up every *"story"* you hear of and correct the (mis)information.
- Remember that it was a *"silly"* comment that, *"**AIDS** is an American **I**deology to **D**iscourage **S**ex"* by the Lobatse students in 1992 that initiated Pictures in AIDucation that thousands have benefited from, in Africa and Europe. Silly has to be replaced by *"powerful"* in this case.
- In the AIDucation workshops, the participants **speak more** than the healthcare workers, facilitators or teachers.
- In the AIDucation workshops, the healthcare workers, facilitators or teachers **learn to listen** as the participants discuss the pictures.
- In the AIDucation workshops, the healthcare workers, facilitators or teachers **build their messages** from the participants' comments and words.

HIVT-F 2: The hidden epidemic

HIV/AIDS – the hidden epidemic

People with AIDS

People with HIV related illness

People with asymptomatic HIV infection

HIVT-F2

ACTSAP:

- Talk about the seriousness of HIV infection and AIDS in the local villages or towns evidenced by the many funerals, sick off notes, orphans, absenteeism at schools and work places
- Talk about the many people being infected but do not know that fact
- Talk about the HIV (antibody) test and NOT the AIDS Test
- Talk about participants going for a voluntary HIV test – *"Know your status."*

TIPS

- No ice-bergs in Africa, so use of hippo for *"tip of the ice-berg"* point.
- Other comparisons used are a crocodile in the water with only its eyes and top of the head showing or a big tree chopped down and submerged in water with only the branches and twigs showing above the surface.
- Message being illustrated and emphasised is of *"a handful"* of people with HIV infection and AIDS that are known or seen or have come out public. The majority of *"healthy looking"* people who are HIV positive and living with HIV infection are not known. A lot of us might be carrying the virus and we do not know it.

- o Mention that if we are sexually active and have not tested for HIV infection, then we cannot say with 100% certainty that we are HIV antibody negative.
- o This is where the danger lies, *"…one cannot tell by looks alone. We might all be HIV positive in this room!"* This statement jolts the participants and gets them thinking as many believe that a person with HIV infection or AIDS is physically *"…finished…wasted…very thin… emaciated…cannot walk…skin on bones… ugly to look at…are greyish black in colour…looks dusty…have baby hair…thin stretched, silky, hair…have a very dry, rough skin…usually cannot breathe properly …have got sores all over the body that do not heal…have no sexual feelings …cannot have an erection…cannot have sex…cannot have babies!"*

Community talks with person living with HIV infection or a *"…Positive Speaker"*

At the end of the first day of the planned three to five days AIDucation course, the Athlone Team would ask a person living with HIV infection to share his or her testimony with the participants. The participants would usually be waiting for the guest speaker, person living with HIV infection, to walk in through the main door. They were visibly shocked and surprised when they saw one of their own – *"normal, healthy looking participant"*- who had registered and checked in with them, in the morning, stand up and come to the front to speak.

He or she would introduce himself or herself, *"…My name is EM. I was diagnosed with HIV infection eight years ago. For those of you who have never seen a person living with HIV, here I am. I notice that I look healthier than some of you in here. It has been a pleasure having this AIDucation session with you and I have also learnt quite a lot!"*

One could literally hear a pin drop in that hall or meeting room, with some faces of the participants still showing shock and utter disbelief. Some participants would even start apologising for their previous comments of *"…these people must be killed otherwise they will infect us all…they are paying the price for their behaviour…people with AIDS are dangerous people…these people must be isolated…AIDS is for prostitutes…these are people who have too many boyfriends or girlfriends…how did the government control the cattle lung disease (implying killing them)?…Government must not waste money looking after these dangerous people…Dr Mapara what do you think you are trying to prove wasting Botswana government money on such a programme?"*

LESSONS LEARNT

1. The lack of knowledge on HIV infection and AIDS out there is frightening.
2. AIDucation is needed in the developing and developed countries as a matter of urgency.

HIVT-F 3: Structure of the human immunodeficiency virus

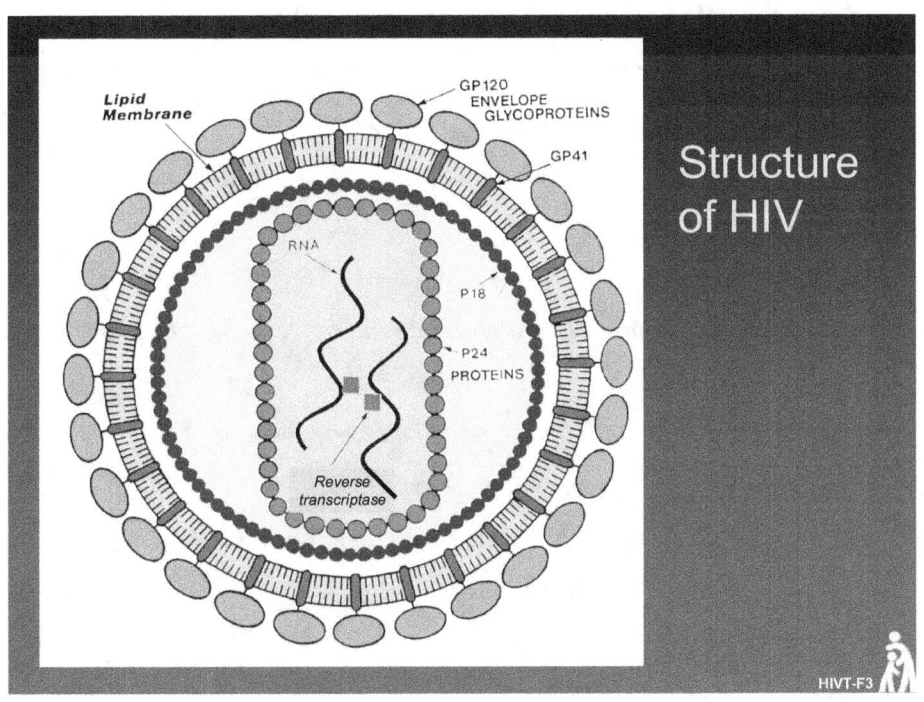

ACTSAP:

- Talk about the cause of HIV infection and AIDS

- Talk about the two types of HIV infections caused by HIV Type 1 and HIV Type 2

- Talk about the local vernacular terms for the virus

- Talk about the fact that HIV infection has no cure.

TIPS

o Talk of HIV Type 1 and HIV Type 2. What are the differences – incubation period, window period, aggressiveness and geographical location?

o The virus is very, very small. HIV cannot be seen with the naked eye or a normal microscope. HIV can only be seen by the help of a very special (electron) microscope.

o Virus described as *"an ant"* or *"insect"* in various vernacular languages.

o Like all viruses, HIV has no cure. Just like a cold or flu has no cure.

o Talk of the changing properties (mutations) of the skin, cover or coat of the virus.

o Talk of the changing properties of the *"internal organs…insides…"* of the virus.

o Compare with TB or fungal infections where the skin, cover, coat and *"internal organs"* remain the same.

- You must state that, "...*This is where the problem is in finding a cure. The changing skin and insides of the virus make it difficult.*"

- There is no cure for HIV infection. There is no cure for AIDS.

- Rub in the fact that there are no traditional (herbs) or western medicines (tablets or injections) that cure HIV infection or AIDS to date.

- The antibiotics or anti-fungal drugs treat bacterial and fungal infections respectively which are "*not changing*" germs.

Community talks about HIV *"behaves like a chameleon"* or *"...a bird that is flying!"*

When discussed in the vernacular or local language, this picture makes a lot of sense to the participants. One participant even commented that, *"This virus behaves like a chameleon – changing colours. Like a chameleon, it hides and one cannot easily see it."*

Another participant commented that, *"It is easier to shoot a bird perched on a tree (TB), than a bird that is flying or is in motion (HIV infection)."*

LESSONS LEARNT

1. Very technical terms and concepts (jargon) can be simplified comfortably into every day language to relay the same scientific message.

2. Patience is a virtue in AIDucation.

3. AIDucation is about shared information, knowledge, dialogue and effective communication.

4. AIDucation is about breaking the loud silence on HIV infection and AIDS in the communities.

HIVT-F 4: The immune system (body defence system)

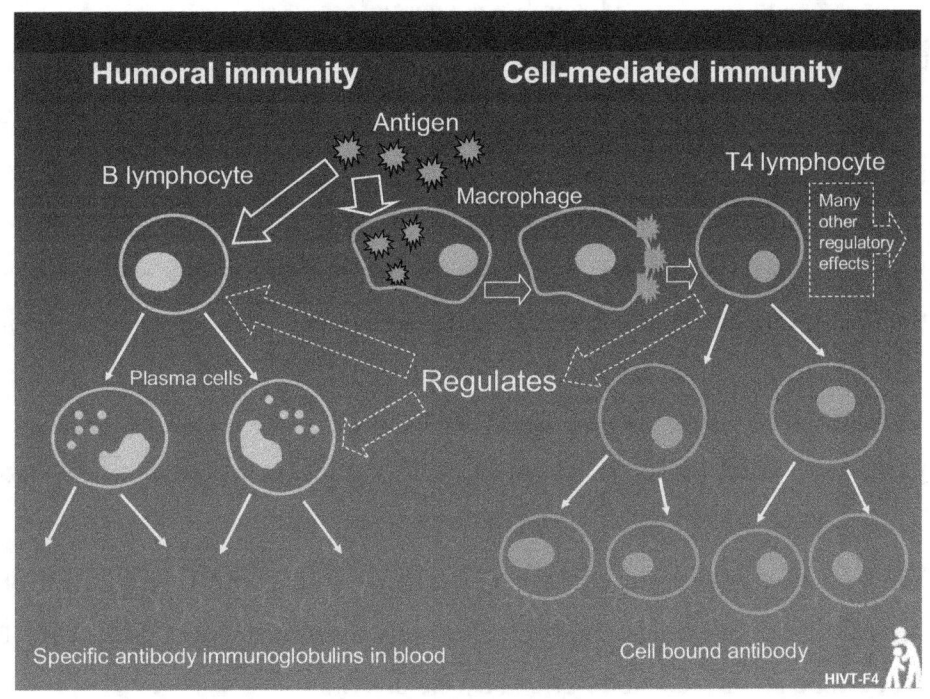

ACTSAP:

- Talk about the body defence system with the two types of *"soldiers from the barracks."*

- Talk about the B soldiers from the "B barracks" and T soldiers from the "T barracks" in the body.

- Talk about how HIV infection weakens the body defence system and eventually causes death by destroying or killing the "B and T soldiers" in the barracks, in the body.

TIPS

- o This is a difficult picture but it can be described in an easy way.

- o The immune system is described in terms of soldiers or the country's defence forces such as the Botswana Defence Forces (BDF) made up of the Special Forces (B- cells) and the regular army (T- cells).

- o What is the role of the army? To defend or protect the country (body) from enemy soldiers.

- o Similarly, the Special Forces (B soldiers) protect the body from Bacterial infections ("Zambian enemy forces").

- The regular army (<u>T</u> soldiers) protects the body from the four enemy forces - <u>T</u>B ("Zimbabwe enemy forces"), fungal infections ("Namibia enemy forces"), viral infections ("South Africa enemy forces") and cancers ("Mozambique enemy forces").

- What happens when the Special Forces and the regular armies are attacked and destroyed?

- The answer is, *"...The BDF is weakened or killed!"* This allows the Zambians, Zimbabweans, Namibians, South Africans and Mozambique enemy forces to enter Botswana.

- These "enemy forces" are now equated to the common infections seen in people living with HIV infection or AIDS clients. Examples of bacterial infections such as abscesses, chest infections and commonly tuberculosis; fungal infections such as ringworms or oral thrush; viral infections such as herpes zoster (shingles) or herpes simplex (cold sores); cancers such as lymphomas or Kaposi's sarcoma which we shall see in the pictures to follow.

- It is these infections or other diseases that kill a person and not HIV infection directly.

- Note the **B** soldiers that protect us from **Bacterial** infections.

- Note the **T** soldiers that protect us from **Tuberculosis, viral and fungal infections.**

- The infections, diseases or cancers that are usually expected when a patient has HIV infection or AIDS, can be predicted and described by the doctors.

Community talks with the national army during outreach talks

During one of Athlone Hospital's outreach programmes to an army barracks, in 1996, one of the soldiers, a Captain, passed an interesting comment after two hours of AIDucation. He said, *"Ngaka (doctor), this is very serious. From what you have described, we have a war on our hands, which is worse than any war that we (soldiers) can go to!"* Little did the Army Captain realise that the President of Botswana, His Excellency Festus Mogae, would declare a war on AIDS in October 2001, when he said, *"Ntwa e boletswe (A war has been declared)!"*

Community talks with a mother of a patient with AIDS

"Thank you for telling us. We guessed that it was AIDS, from what you have been teaching us in the village. It is a burden off our shoulders, knowing the truth. Thank you." This was the response from a mother of a patient with AIDS that the nurses failed to break the *"bad news"* to for fear of *"...depressing her and hurting her."* The truth will always set us free. It is hard enough for the relatives to nurse a dying patient, but they must be told the truth. There is no shame in dying of AIDS. Often as healthcare workers we fear the unknown. We fear our own fears and place them on others.

105

HIVT-F 5: How HIV infects T4 cells

How HIV infects T4 cells

VIRUS
CD4 receptor molecule
T4 CELL CYTOPLASM
Enters host cell, loses envelope
RT enzyme
NUCLEUS
Viral RNA
T4 cell genome
RNA DNA
copies of viral RNA (messenger RNA)
Viral DNA
New viruses bud out of T4 cell
viral genome integrates with T4 cell genome
HIVT-F5

ACTSAP

- Talk about how HIV enters the body's soldiers and destroys them

- Talk about the soldiers of the body as "houses" that HIV enters

- Reassure participants not to worry if they do not understand this picture. It is not a simple one.

TIPS

- o This is another busy, complex picture. The participants usually open their mouths wide in awe or despair. Reassure them.

- o This picture is made easy, by asking the participants to shut their eyes and imagine a visitor (HIV) coming to visit you at your house (body soldier). The visitor knocks on the door (body soldier's door) of the house.

- o The door of the house is opened as you answer, *"Tsena… karibu…(come in!)"*

- o The visitor takes off the jacket or coat and leaves it outside on a coat hanger. The visitor enters the house and heads for the master bedroom (nucleus or engine to go and sleep or have sex with you / your engine).

- o You and the visitor have sexual intercourse and a chain of babies are produced.

o Note that to get to the bedroom, the visitor (HIV) has to cross the sitting room carpet or shower (reverse transcriptase enzyme) that washes it and makes it sexually excited. Sexual intercourse takes place in the master bedroom. Sex leads to pregnancy. Chains of babies are formed. The chains must be cut up to release the baby viruses to go out through the doors and windows. This is done by a scissors (protease enzyme).

o A bit of information on how antiretroviral therapy works is discussed – stopping or blocking carpet movement or shower (reverse transcriptase inhibitor) and scissors cutting action (Protease inhibitor).

o Groups of drugs are reverse transcriptase inhibitors and protease inhibitors.

o There are now other groups of drugs on the market, including those that block at the "door" so that HIV does not enter the "house" to cause damage.

o Many participants, especially those on anti-HIV drugs love and appreciate this illustration.

Community talks on "...*changing nature*" of the virus called HIV

Many participants have commented that;

o *"I did not know that these drugs work like a lock and key!"*

o *"I did not know that these drugs work at different sites and have a special function. I was selecting which drugs to drink, like I used to do when taking high blood pressure tablets. Now I will not after what I have learnt."*

o *"To kill the virus means killing a part of the person."*

o *"Taking the drugs is like stepping on the head of a snake. You do not lift your foot off the head of the snake if you want to survive. You know what happens if you lift your foot!"*

o *"Taking these drugs is like a marriage, but with no room for divorce!"*

o *"Many clients are selective on taking treatment. They know which drugs cause terrible side-effects, so they leave them out. This leads to drug resistant HIV strains!"*

o *"This is AIDS made easy!"*...*"These doctors do not explain these actions to us!"*

LESSONS LEARNT

- The lack of knowledge on how antiretroviral therapy or the anti-HIV drugs work is a major factor for the clients missing out drugs or selecting which drugs to drink.

- Do not assume that these pictures are too difficult for lay people to understand.

HIVT-F 6: HIV inside the T4 cell

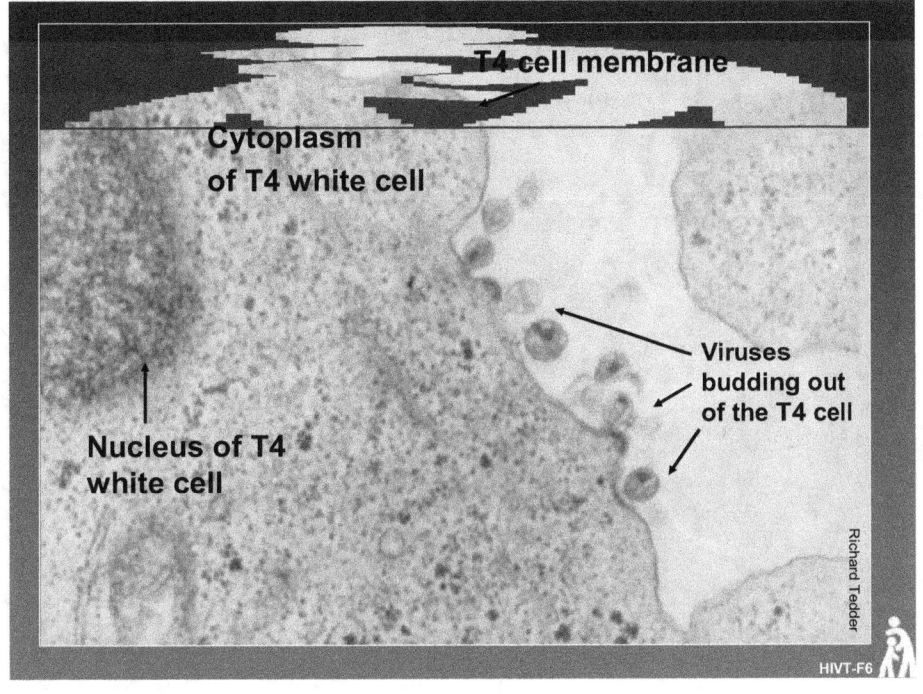

ACTSAP

- Talk about how the real HIV babies look like when coming out of the T4 cell or house, as seen in this picture, where the HIV babies are holding onto the *"doors"* and *"windows"* and preparing to move on after putting on their coats.

- Compare the *"real"* microscope picture of HIV and the previous diagram of HIV taking off its coat and entering the house, having sex and the babies being born. Recall the HIV babies coming out, leaving the cell or house and putting on their coats to attack other soldiers (houses).

TIPS

- ○ Challenging picture to describe.
- ○ Small explanation of the viruses or *"germs"* or *"insects"* as seen by a special microscope.
- ○ Explain the picture in terms of *"soap bubbles (baby viruses)"* coming out from a squeezed soap or detergent bottle (the T-soldier or the house)."
- ○ Visuals, imagination, use of day-to-day words and materials play an important role in Pictures in AIDucation. *"Seeing is very different from being told."*

HIVT - F7: Natural history of HIV infection

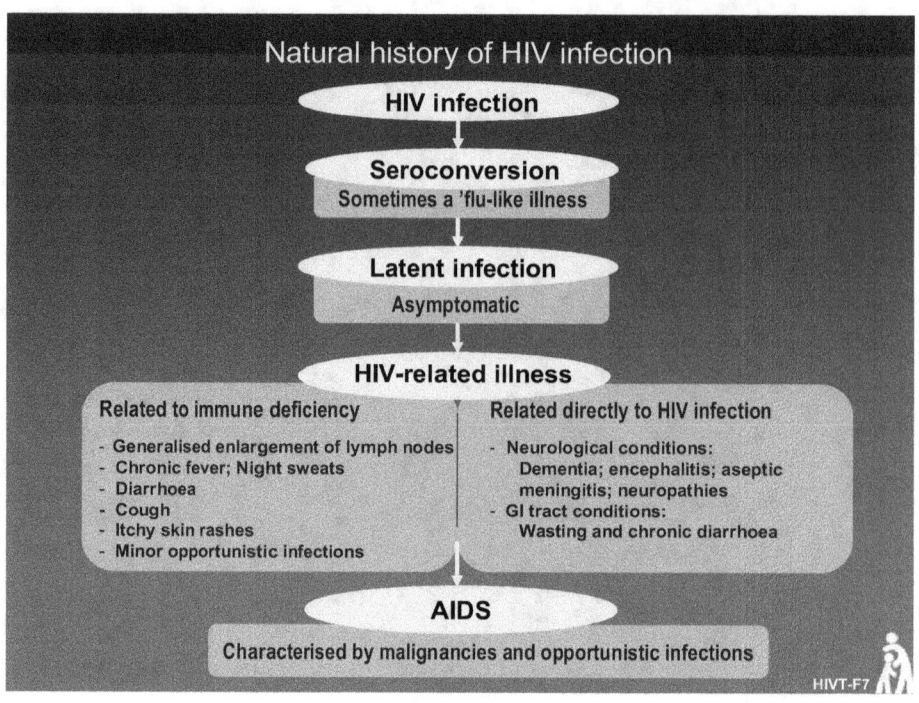

ACTSAP

- Talk a little bit about the medical jargon in the slide and try to simplify it into "normal" everyday English or into the vernacular language that can be understood

- Talk about some of the ways that people with HIV infection might present at the clinic or show illness or disease

- Talk about what HIV infection, the beginning of infection and the difference with AIDS, the advanced stage or full-blown picture.

TIPS

- Summarise the possible stages and outcomes of HIV infection.

- Talk about HIV infection from beginning to *"carrier state"* to full-blown AIDS.

- Ensure that participants understand that HIV infection and AIDS are not the same. These are TWO different diseases or conditions.

- Define the scientific words *sero-conversion, window period, latent (hidden)* infections in the most basic sentences.

- To make matters easier, I usually talk of myself engaging in unprotected sex with a person living with HIV infection or a *"you me nice (commercial sex worker or prostitute),"* as called

109

in the local Botswana slang. I would then go on to describe the steps that I would go through to develop HIV infection and years later develop full blown AIDS. At times I talk of myself as if I am HIV positive or living with HIV infection and passing on the virus, sexually, to one of the female participants. We then discuss the stages that the female participant will go through to becoming HIV infected and years later developing AIDS.

o State that not all patients who have HIV infection will develop AIDS. A very small proportion of people do not develop AIDS.

o The majority of HIV infected clients later became very ill and develop AIDS.

o There are those clients we call *rapid progressors* and *slow progressors* in terms of developing AIDS. This fact or statement gives hope of long life, to those who wrongly believe that HIV infection is "*instant death...a death sentence.*"

o Remember "*Hope Is Vital (HIV)*" when living with the human immunodeficiency virus (HIV) in the body.

o Talk about "*discordant couples*" where one partner is HIV positive and the other is HIV negative despite the couple having unprotected sex for years. It is not automatic that if one partner is HIV positive then the other will be HIV positive. That is the reason for each individual to do an HIV test – "*know your status.*" You cannot depend on your partner's HIV positive or negative result to state your HIV status.

o Go for your own voluntary HIV test. It is important to do so if you love yourself and if you love those around you.

Community talks on medical language (jargon)

An AIDucation workshop participant said, "*Many doctors and nurses forget that we do not know these long, difficult words of yours. When you ask them to explain, they even give you more difficult words and explanations. They must teach with pictures like you do, so that we can see for ourselves what they are trying to tell us. Sometimes they become angry because you are wasting their time and they tell you that they have too many other patients to see. The traditional doctors do not rush you. They are patient and they listen to you. The traditional doctors treat you like a person.*"

LESSONS LEARNT

1. Be patient with the clients.

2. Keep it short and simple (KISS) when talking to clients.

3. The traditional doctors seem to be good counsellors and have a holistic approach to disease.

HIVT - F8: Viral load and the immune system response

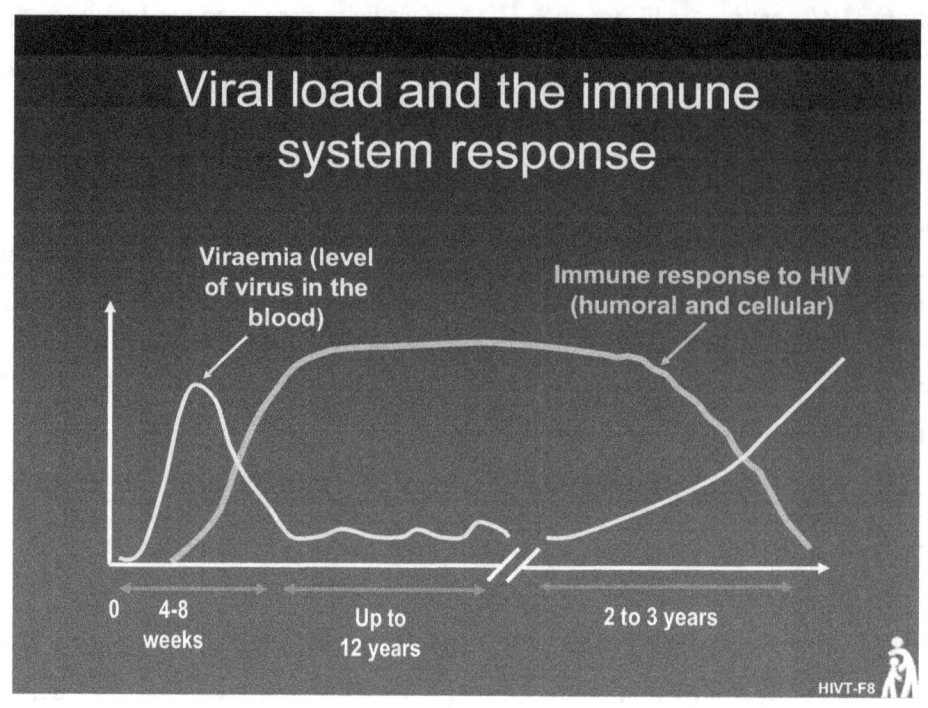

ACTSAP

- Talk about the meaning of the term *"viral load"* or concentration of the virus in the body

- Talk about the normal "soldiers (CD4 cells)" in the body and how they respond to the presence of HIV infection

- Talk about how healthcare workers use viral load and the CD4 cell count to see or monitor how a person on treatment, antiretroviral therapy, is responding.

TIPS

- Not necessary to explain graph, but might depend on level of education of participants.

- Simple definition of viral load or concentration or amount of the virus in the body.

- Simple definition of CD4 (body soldiers) using the normal "Western" levels of 500 – 1500 soldiers in the barracks, although these can vary remarkably in Africans and tend to be lower.

- Relationship between viral load and CD4.

- When client is on treatment and responds well to the anti-HIV drugs the viral load goes down, while the CD4 count increases or the *"soldiers in the barracks"* multiply.

- If patient is not responding well to treatment or not taking medication as prescribed, the viral load goes up and the CD4 goes down or the *"soldiers in the barracks"* reduce in numbers.

o There is no cure for HIV infection or AIDS to date. The CD4 count is also used to understand the general state of health of the client or patient living with HIV infection or AIDS.

o Discuss the possible causes of viral load going up and CD4 coming down when client is on treatment to emphasise need for taking treatment religiously and at the exact times prescribed.

o Some Positive Speakers are able to discuss the CD4 and viral load very well, using their real life experiences. Work with people living with HIV infection and AIDS, they are generally under-utilised teachers, facilitators, adherence counsellors and consultants.

Community talks on *"undetectable levels"* of HIV in the body

A young 16 year old girl who was diagnosed HIV positive went around the village telling the community members that she had been *"...cured from AIDS"* according to the private doctor who had told her that *"...the virus was undetectable...and I am doing well!"* The young lady had not understood what the doctor had said to her. The doctor, when contacted, said that he thought that the young lady had understood what he had told her. There had been a communication breakdown.

The young lady was later contacted by one of the hospital counsellors and they had a discussion on her HIV status. The counsellor talked to her about HIV infection and AIDS and the meaning of the various blood tests that are usually done. The counsellor went on to explain the meaning of the term *"undetectable levels."* The client was disappointed but went away AIDucated and empowered. She was still HIV positive, infectious and responding well to treatment.

Community talks about *"...I am bisexual"* when meant heterosexual or *"straight"*

A man came in for an HIV test. On taking his details, he said that he was *"bisexual"* without any inhibitions or embarrassment. I asked the gentleman to explain what he meant by *"bisexual"* as he was bisexual. He happily responded, as he raised two fingers, stressing the *"bi"* as in two. *"I just have sex with my wife, just the two of us,"* he responded.

I explained the meaning of the word bisexual. He cried, *"God forbid! I do not have sex with men!"* To make matters worse, he had been filling *"bisexual"* in all the legal documents that needed personal detail and had asked on sexuality.

LESSONS LEARNT

1. Be clear with those medical terms and explanations.
2. Do not assume that we all understand *"undetectable levels (Absent?)"* or *"bisexual (two?)"* or *"status (immigration?)"* that might have ambiguous or double meanings.

HIVT – F9: HIV antibody testing – ELISA

ACTSAP

- Talk about the types of HIV antibody tests performed in the local hospital, clinic or voluntary counselling and testing centres

- Talk about the length of time it takes to perform the HIV tests and the reasons for the delay or early test results

- Talk about the blood transfusion services and what types of tests (HIV test, hepatitis test, syphilis, sickle cell disease) that they do when the blood bank team collects blood donations from blood donors in the community.

TIPS

- Ask for volunteers to share their experiences on donating blood.
- Ask for volunteers to share their experiences on HIV antibody tests done and the reason for the HIV tests that they did. No need to give out HIV test results, unless the person has been prepared to go public or is a known trained "Positive Speaker" from a support group.
- Discuss pre-test counselling and post-test counselling briefly.
- Emphasise the need for permission and a signed, informed consent for an HIV test.

Community talks on "...test for everything"

An elderly lady, in her sixties, had lost her husband to AIDS when she was about forty-five years old. The woman was relatively healthy until, almost fifteen years later, when she began to lose weight and cough. She had gone to see her doctor at the clinic and told the doctor to "...*test me for everything.*" The tests were done and "...*nothing was found*" according to her. She came to see me at the clinic, tired of being told that she was okay when she knew that there was something "...*not right.*" After talking to her about the possible causes of her illness, she agreed and consented for an HIV test. The test was done after pre-test counselling. She was found to be HIV positive. She had "...*expected it*" but was very disappointed that she had seen her local doctor five times and five times her doctor had said, "...*the blood tests are fine*" and according to her interpretation. "...*I had no AIDS.*" She complained bitterly, saying, "*I told him to test for everything!*" She had wanted the HIV test to be done and had wrongly assumed that it was part of the "...*test for everything.*"

On my making a follow-up with the doctor, he told me that, "...*she did not seem to be in the age group for HIV infection or AIDS*" and therefore did not think of an HIV test on her.

LESSONS LEARNT

1. The client or patient should specifically request for an HIV test and not to request for "...*test for everything.*"

2. No age group is exempt from HIV infection or AIDS. The oldest person I know that is living with HIV infection is about seventy years old, fit and active. He is not on treatment. He is on "...*a second life from God*" according to him and smiles comfortably saying "... *my secret is a healthy diet from God's soil. Not from the factories...I take each day as it comes and thank God for each day's blessings!*"

3. Encourage sexually active people to have an HIV test. They have more to gain than to lose.

4. Young men and women can acquire sexually transmitted infections, including HIV infection or AIDS.

5. Elderly men and women can acquire sexually transmitted infections, including HIV infection and AIDS.

6. AIDucation is about raising awareness on HIV infection, AIDS and encouraging HIV testing.

HIVT – F10: Rapid/simple tests

ACTSAP

- Talk about the rapid or simple tests and how they are done or performed

- Talk about the colour changes seen in these small wells or pots and the meanings of the various colour changes

- Talk about the tests performed at your local hospital, clinic or voluntary counselling and testing centre.

TIPS

o Rapid HIV antibody tests in some centres are done within 15-20 minutes.

o Explain the full test procedure to the client.

o I usually explain the finger prick test to the client so that the client will tell me the test result after 15 or 20 minutes. This change of role is about the client owning the results. It is about the client being empowered. It is about the client informing others.

o Explain what a positive result means and what a negative result means.

o Pre and post test counselling are very important.

o Remember issues of confidentiality.

o Ask a laboratory technician or officer from the voluntary counselling and testing centre to explain HIV antibody tests. They are happy to discuss their services with you.

Community talks on *"betrayal"* by faith leader(s)

A God fearing young lady living with HIV infection was forced to leave her church, where she had grown up and worshipped for many years, after she was *"... betrayed"* by her pastor. After three years of quietly living with her HIV positive diagnosis, she told the pastor in confidence about her HIV status. The pastor was *"...very understanding"* and told her that he would remember her in his prayers. She went away happy and comforted, *"...having shared my burden with my pastor."*

The following Sunday was a *"...nightmare, I will never forget"* she told me. *"The pastor told the church congregation of close to 600 members that I had AIDS and they should all pray for me. He even told me to stop taking the treatment, as God would perform a miracle on me and heal me, through faith."* The lady broke down, as she talked of how all of a sudden she had lost all her friends and how the world had *"...turned upside down."* Worse still she was now called *"...a prostitute"* by her own relatives despite having known *"...only one man in my life!"*

She later moved to a different town *"...to start life all over again."* She did not make *"...the mistake of telling my new pastor."* She has continued taking her treatment and remains very positive about the future *"...taking each day as it comes and thanking God for the gift of life."*

The man of God had wrecked the woman's life (un)intentionally. The church has to be compassionate when dealing with its flock that is living with HIV infection or AIDS in the church. No one is immune to HIV infection, including pastors, as the African Network of Religious Leaders living with HIV infection and AIDS (ANERELA+) has shown. ANERELA+ is comprised of men and women of the collar, pastors, deacons, church elders and Imams who are HIV positive or are affected by HIV infection and AIDS.

LESSONS LEARNT

1. One should think twice about whom to tell or share or disclose their HIV status.
2. Confidentiality must be respected.
3. Faith leaders or faith communities must not stop any hospital prescribed treatment for patients – be it treatment for pain, asthma, diabetes, hypertension, HIV infection or AIDS.
4. Prayers and medical treatment go together.
5. The faith communities and healthcare workers work together in AIDucation.
6. The faith communities need Pastoral AIDucation. Amen.

HIVT – 11: HIV antibody test results and the window period

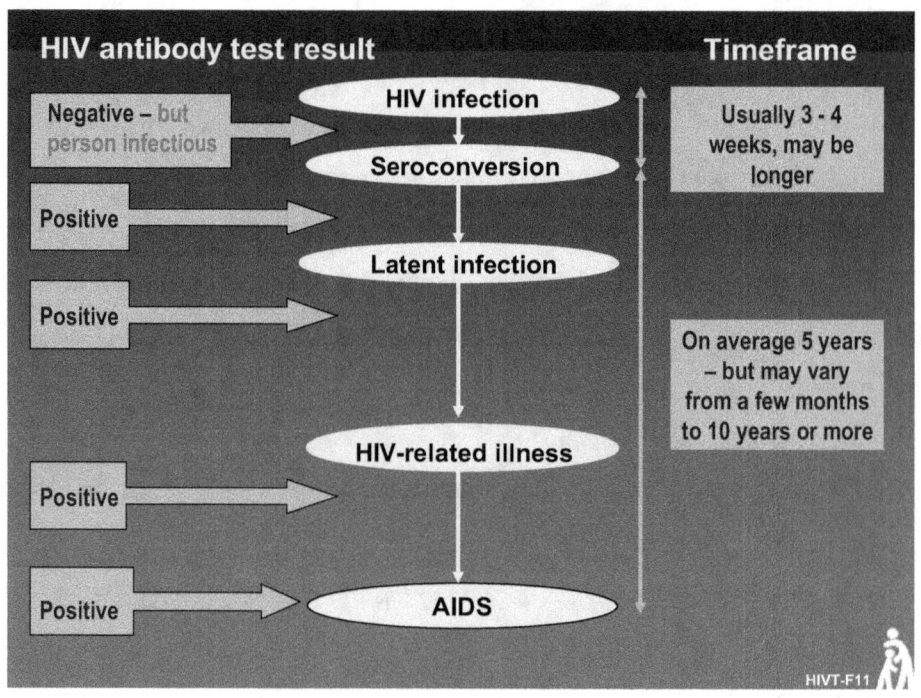

ACTSAP

These three "technical" slides, F9, F10 and F11 on HIV antibody testing are discussed together. Do not leave them out because they look complicated. You can seek assistance and call in the laboratory technician or the counsellor/officer from the voluntary counselling and testing centre to come and help talk about the HIV antibody tests or screening.

- Talk about why we need (reasons) to have an HIV test done

- Talk about the process of having an HIV test done

- Talk about what is expected in terms of colour changes when the HIV test is done or the meaning of the red line(s) seen on the rapid test strip after the HIV finger-prick test.

TIPS

- o Very basic information on the types of HIV tests or test kits used by your local clinic, hospital or voluntary counselling and testing centre.

- o Talk briefly about informed consent and confidentiality. Never get tired of repeating these basic facts.

- Give a few reasons for having the HIV test done, such as hospital or personal reasons. All voluntary HIV tests must have pre-test counselling and signed consent for the HIV test to be performed.
- Some reasons for HIV testing include:
  - Where a medical diagnosis has to be made
  - Screening for blood transfusions
  - When patient has tuberculosis (TB), herpes zoster (shingles), chicken-pox in adults, Kaposi's sarcoma, chronic fever, chronic diarrhoea and general body swellings
  - When patient has a sexually transmitted infection, especially where there are ulcers
  - Before marriage, before pregnancy or during pregnancy
  - Simply to *"know your HIV status"* which is being encouraged by many countries
  - Patients are admitted in the hospital. Routine "opt-out" HIV tests for all patients being admitted in the hospital are being encouraged.

Community talks on *"…suicides"* in the early days of the epidemics

A man committed suicide because he believed that he was *"HIV Positive"* and his doctor was *"…hiding this fact"* from him, according to the suicide note that he left behind. His out-patient card showed that he was *"VDRL POSITIVE"* and this result was written in red ink by his doctor. The man had syphilis, another type of sexually transmitted infection that has treatment and can be cured. The man took his life out of ignorance, believing that he was *"HIV POSITIVE."*

Many people during the early days of the epidemic committed suicide on being told that they were HIV positive, because of lack of knowledge and good information. This should not happen in this day and era. An HIV positive result is not *"…an automatic death sentence."* HIV infection is a chronic infection and not necessarily a fatal disease or illness. Living positively (healthy) with HIV infection can prolong life and delay the development of AIDS.

LESSONS LEARNT

1. Write the details of the patient on the out-patient department (OPD) card with caution. The red ink or block letters or capital letters for emphasis might not be a very good idea.
2. The word "POSITIVE" must be explained clearly whatever the test is that is being done or carried out. The words *"positive"* and *"counselling"* are somehow usually associated with HIV infection and AIDS in most cases.

HIVT – F12: Genetic variability of the virus

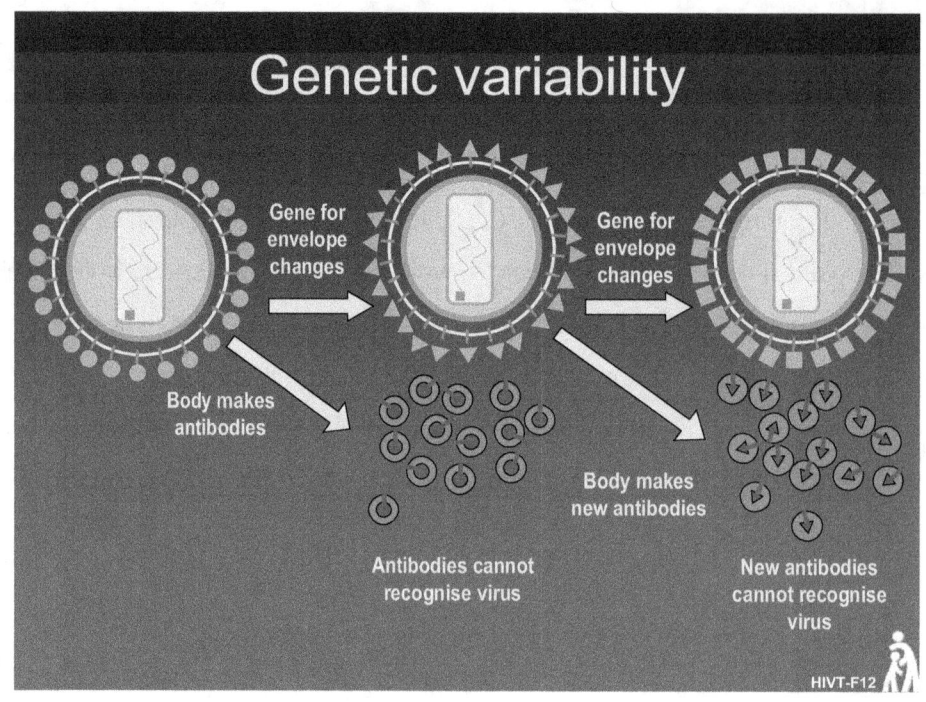

ACTSAP

- Talk about the changing *"coat"* or *"skin"* and *"insides"* of the virus

- Talk about the difficulties of discovering a cure because of this changing property or behaviour of HIV

- Talk about how the *"coat"* or *"skin"* and *"insides"* remain the same for bacteria causing infections, such as tuberculosis, abscesses, pneumonias or tonsillitis.

TIPS

- Strangely, this is one of the most remembered pictures by the AIDucation workshop participants, the changing coat – from circles to triangles to squares.

- The changing coat of the virus. This picture emphasises the lock (HIV) and key (Drug) mechanism or action. The drug has to bind on the coat of HIV to enter it and kill it, but HIV keeps on changing, so that drug cannot bind or lock on to it. I replace antibodies by drugs.

- Participants who have grasped the basic facts about HIV comment about the changing property of the virus in comparison to TB from the earlier pictures.

119

- Emphasise the need for early HIV antibody testing so as to treat TB if client has both HIV infection and TB. More than 70% of patients in Zambia and Botswana had both HIV and TB combined. TB has a cure.
- HIV infection can be prevented. TB can be cured. AIDS can be stopped.

Community talks on a *"…too clever"* HIV infection and AIDS virus

AIDucation participant said, *"Ngaka (Doctor), I do not see you people getting a cure for AIDS from what you have pictured to us. This virus is too clever for the scientists. It is smart and it thinks like a human being! It is better we prevent the young ones from catching it. Prevention is better than cure."*

Almost twenty years ago, when I first saw this picture, I knew that there was big trouble ahead. It is not rocket science to understand this fact. I was called *"…a pessimist of a junior doctor"* and *"…an alarmist"* for saying that a cure would not be found in the next twenty years, when I was *"… not a scientist!"* Twenty years have almost passed. It will be twenty years in 2009, since I made that *"…alarmist"* statement. I should not say too much until after 2009.

Do I see a cure or a vaccine in the next twenty years, after 2009? I will answer that question after 2009, although not much has changed from my original statement. If anything Pictures in AIDucation is the route to go, if we are going to prevent new HIV infections and avoidable deaths.

Back to the basics as we have been told in public health, *"Prevention is better than cure."*

LESSONS LEARNT

1. *"Genetic variability"* of the virus called HIV is one of the simplest pictures for the grassroots folks. *"Simply the changing skin of the virus"* which is nicely pictured. The message of mutations, without mentioning mutations, is home and dry.
2. Many external evaluators of AIDucation fall into the trap and wonder how anyone in his right senses can talk to traditional doctors about *"Genetic variability"* in an AIDucation session. Ask the traditional doctors in Lobatse, Botswana to explain genetic variability. You will be wonderfully surprised at the depth of knowledge.
3. AIDucation is about faith communities, spiritual support, prayers, emotional support and compassion. AIDucation is about empowerment.
4. AIDucation is about *"Prevention is better than cure!"*
5. Never get tired of talking, teaching and singing about HIV infection and AIDS.

HIVT – F13: Transmission of HIV infection through sex

ACTSAP

- Talk about sexual intercourse and the types of sexual intercourse
- Talk about culture in relation to sexual activities
- Talk about faith communities and sex education
- Talk about who is supposed to teach the young people on sexual intercourse and relationships.

TIPS

o Simply, *"Let us freely talk about sex!"*

o Popular picture of (a) commercial sex worker involved in a condom promotion programme and a client (b) Young peer educators.

o Participants fail to stop talking when they get started on talking about sex. Even the shy, quiet ones get very involved. As one participant said, *"Sex is good, but at the right time and with the right partner. It is a beautiful, but embarrassing subject."*

o These pictures alone can *"talk"* for more than an hour.

o A lot of traditional and cultural issues are discussed because of this picture:

   o Vaginal sex

   o Anal sex *"...homosexuality"* are hot points for discussions. Emotions tend to rise.

o Sexual health promotion in some African countries does not talk or emphasise facts about anal sex or homosexuality, as homosexuality is believed to be *"...Western and for the white people."* This definitely is not true. There are many African gay men and also African lesbians. This is a missed opportunity in Africa. There are homosexual communities in both the developed and developing countries.

o Homosexuality. Usually "very touchy" subject. Homosexuality is present in Africa but the authorities play it down, apart from South Africa that has a big homosexual movement.

o Men having sex with men (MSM) are there. The *"normal or straight"* African man and woman cannot understand how and why men have sex with men and women with women. A very sensitive issue.

o Bi-sexual men. Some men are married, have a wife and children so as to please the parents who want the *"...traditional family name to be passed on to the next generation."* The man also has a male sexual partner. In many cases the wife might not know this hidden fact.

o Bi-sexual women. Some women have sex with both men and women. There is normal penis in vagina sexual intercourse. In some cases all kinds of *"adult toys"* are used when women have sex with women (lesbians).

o Oral sex is *"...not African...it is a sickness...it is not sex..."* say some African folks. Who sets sexual intercourse standards? What is *"...normal"* or *"...abnormal"* sex?

o Use of herbs or traditional medicines to dry and tighten the vagina for *"...tighter and better sex!"* This is reported to be common in Southern Africa where sex is preferred *"dry"* as compared to the north where sex is preferred *"wet"*. Is this true?

o Dry sex predisposes to possible sexually transmitted infections including HIV infection as a result of bruising or cuts in the wall of the dry vagina.

o Sexual intercourse is usually *"...to please the man"* say the elderly women at initiation camps of girls who have come of age. African women are socialised to *"...please your husband. Anytime he demands sex, you give it to him!"* There is usually *"...no refusal of sex in an African marriage."* It is also believed that there is *"no rape"* in an African marriage. It is the, *"...bwana's (sir's) entitlement or parcel!"*

o Participants must be taught about domestic violence and rape in marriages and to speak against these evils. There is no excuse. Couple's must be encouraged to talk about sex freely to each other and to understand each other's sexual needs.

- Both male and female circumcisions are discussed. Beliefs or reasons on why the procedures are done, the meanings and implications are discussed.
- Usually the participants are able to give reasons on why circumcisions are done
- Myths such as *"...sleeping with virgins or young girls cures the HIV infection in the body"* are addressed and discarded. SLEEPING WITH VIRGINS OR YOUNG GIRLS DOES NOT CURE AIDS!

Community talks on *"...oral what?!"*

An elderly female participant in a workshop was shocked, disgusted and very concerned as she asked, *"...Oral what?! What are you children doing eating vaginas and penises? Is it any wonder that we have these incurable diseases! The world is finished! Lord have mercy on these children!"*

Many conservative African families, especially the older generation, cannot imagine *"...going south"*, another term for oral sex, and doing it would be *"...dirty, filthy and plain disgusting."* It is unimaginable. It is a taboo.

One church elder spoke with anger, *"It is abuse of the vagina or penis. God did not create them (genitals) for putting them in the mouth! This generation needs prayers! Stop this evil discussion!"* We stopped... for the day.

Community talks on *"...blow job"* in sexual intercourse

A 13 year old girl came to the out-patient department with a complaint of a *"...headache"*, which was not very convincing. After a bit of prodding and edging on, the girl showed her tongue. She had a syphilitic ulcer (chancre) or a sore of syphilis, a sexually transmitted infection, on the side of the tongue. On further questioning, she said that she had done a *"blow job"* on an elderly man. The nurse I was with in the consulting room did not know what a *"blow job"* was.

Learn the language of the youth or young people if you are going to talk to them on any health matter, including sexual intercourse and relationships. The youth in the borough of Brent, in England, have taught me quite a few sexual terms such as *"...bushing, snowballing, links, daisy-chain, commando, tea-bagging, shiners, bowing, six-nine, London bridge, swinging and swingers' clubs."*

LESSONS LEARNT

- Learn the sexual culture(s) of the community.
- Work together to change the bad sexual practices that spread sexually transmitted infections.
- AIDucation is about enjoying the gift of life, with responsibility, to avoid HIV infection.

HIVT – F14: Sexually transmitted infections increase HIV risk

STIs increase transmission of HIV

Chancroid

Holmes

HIVT-F14

ACTSAP

- Talk about other sexually transmitted infections, especially those with ulcers, sores or open wounds in relation to increasing the risk of catching or contracting HIV infection

- Talk about the importance of seeking proper early treatment at the local health facility and not buying treatment over the counter or in chemists without a proper prescription from the doctors or nurses.

TIPS

o Mention that there are more than 26 types of sexually transmitted infections.

o Give a broad classification or groups of these infections – bacterial, fungal, parasitic and viral. Give an example of each, using the local or vernacular words where possible. No need for details.

o Chancroid ulcer discussed in relation to other sexually transmitted infections with ulcers such as syphilis or herpes infections.

o Chancroid is also present in England. I mention it here as one UK doctor in one of my AIDucation sessions in England almost convinced us that there was no chancroid in the England, saying that, *"Chancroid is only found in Africa."*

- Entry point of HIV infection on *"...that door (wound) on the shaft of the penis."*

- This picture opens up frank talk and helps to reduce embarrassment.

- Many participants find it hard to believe that some sexually transmitted infections like syphilis are not painful and ask, *"How is it possible to have such a large wound (syphilis) and not feel the pain?"*

- Then the issue of looking at and inspecting the partner's penis or vagina before intercourse is brought in.

- On telling the participants to look at their partners' sexual organs next time they have sex, there would often be an outcry! *"...It raises suspicion ...one is questioning the faithfulness of the partner...the manhood (penis) and womanhood (vagina) are not for looking at...it would be hard for me to examine the man's penis... I just cannot look at it!"*

- Many women say it would be difficult to show their partners their vaginas out of embarrassment. As one lady said, *"I just cannot! Apart from being embarrassing, God made it and covered it. It is not for public shows. It must remain covered, hidden and respected!"*

One can see the difficulties of talking about sex and relationships in these AIDucation workshops, but we have no choice. We have to talk about sex or else we will keep on counting the ever increasing new sexually transmitted infections including HIV infections, deaths and experiencing the hardships brought about by HIV infection and AIDS.

Community talks on nudity

One elderly woman who had been married for almost 15 years said, *"I have never seen the bwana's (sir's) manhood!"* *"What of when bathing or showering together?"* I asked. She replied, *"...bathing with who? It is not possible!"* She had never bathed or showered with her husband before. I continued with my questions, *"What of when undressing?"* She replied, *"It is done under the bed-sheets and in the dark!"* I resisted from talking with her about fore-play lest I was taken before the elders and charged for being *"disrespectful."*

Community talks about talking about monthly periods

On the issue of talking about sex with the partner, one participant said, *"...It does not happen. There is no discussion. If he wants the parcel, I give it to him!"* *"What of talking about the monthly periods?"* I enquire. *"It is taboo! In my culture, when I am at the moon (monthly period) I put a white handkerchief on the dressing table or on my side of the headboard for my husband to see and he understands that I am not well!"* Other women use *"…traditional waist beads"* or a *"…special cloth"* placed strategically for the sexual partner to understand.

In other cultures, when the woman is having her monthly periods, she does not cook in those three or four days during the periods. Other women cook but do not put salt in the food being cooked and call upon one of the children to put in the salt. Some children ask about why they are being sent to put salt in the food. The reasons given are anything else apart from talking about the mother's or sister's monthly periods.

LESSONS LEARNT

1. We have to talk more on sexually transmitted infections at home, the schools, workplaces, churches and various community associations. It is an embarrassing subject, but we have no choice.

2. *"Culture, Sex and Religion"* must be a topic for discussion if we are going to address or contain the spread of sexually transmitted infections.

3. AIDucation is about self-respect and mutual respect.

4. AIDucation is more than World AIDS Day.

5. AIDucation is about living with HIV infections and AIDS in the community every single day.

HIVT-F15: Mobility increases risk of HIV infection

ACTSAP

- Talk about mobile populations or people on the move (that is all of us) and what could happen on the journey or towards the end of the journey in terms of sexual relationships
- Talk about who is to blame for HIV infection and AIDS in your country
- Talk about all of us being at risk and to blame, so long as we are sexually active.

TIPS

- This picture is a *"...an exciting workshop"* by itself and generates all kinds of comments, discussions and stories. Who is to blame?
- We are all to blame for today's HIV infection and AIDS situation in the world, by our action or inaction.
- *"Men behaving badly"* and *"women behaving badly"* stories are abundant.
- Mobility reported as a cause of HIV infection amongst women as *"...many wives are infected by their husbands who travel on business trips."*
- *"Some women on across border businesses would rather pay with their bodies rather than part with the hard earned "forex (foreign currency)."*

o *"It is known that some women who go to buy fish at the lakes or rivers have marriages of convenience at the fish camps."*

o *"Men drive trucks and men drive AIDS. They bring AIDS into the home. They transport AIDS. When he dies, his relatives blame us (women) for giving him AIDS!"*

o *"Now small girls are having sex with men older than their fathers. Shamuna (shame)!"*

o *"These young boys are undressing women old enough to be their mothers! What has happened to this world? These are the days of Sodoma (Sodom) and Gomorrah!"*

Community talks on *"…separation of spouses"* in the civil service

An AIDucation participant said, *"…Talk to the government to review its policy (General Orders) about separation of spouses. In other countries people get married to live together, but in this country (Botswana), married couples can be separated by the government to work at different ends of the country, as their services are needed by all Batswana. This leads to men getting a second wife or owning a 'ntlo nyana (small house)' and this leads to the spread of AIDS."*

Community talks on men's emotions … *"he wants sex!"*

One elderly man stood up, in a neighbouring village, after an AIDucation session with the Athlone team. There was silence as he cleared his throat to speak and for attention. *"Ngaka, you and your team have got a very difficult task. I do not envy you. If this AIDS was acquired through a different route like coughing or shaking of hands you would have a chance to stop it. Now we know that this AIDS is caught mainly through thobalo (sex), which man cannot do without."*

He went on to explain why it was difficult, as he thoughtfully and pensively looked around the room. *"Ngaka, when a man is happy, he wants sex."* He paused for the message to sink in. He continued, *"When a man is sad he wants sex."* He paused again, taking his time, *"When a man is drunk he wants sex, even though he cannot do the job."* The old man continued driving the sexual points and lessons home, *"When a man is angry and frustrated he wants sex… When a man has been promoted at work he wants sex… When a man has been fired at work he wants sex… When a man is stressed he wants sex…When a man wants entertainment, he wants sex."* The old man paused, fixed his eyes on a group of young men in the audience and continued, looking in their direction, *"You had better talk to these young men who think that the world revolves between their legs. They will perish if they do not think higher than their waists!"*

The old man sat down as the other elders nodded their heads in approval of the words of the peer, the words of wisdom. Meanwhile the young men were smiling and giggling mischievously.

128

HIVT-F16: Transmission of HIV through blood

ACTSAP

- Talk about HIV transmission or spread through unscreened blood transfusions, through contaminated, dirty needles, syringes, blades or surgical equipment
- Talk about HIV transmission through razor blades used by the traditional doctors for scarification marks
- Talk about the importance of blood donations to save life.

TIPS

- These pictures are AIDucation workshops on their own.
- Blood transfusions or donations are used for saving lives. Always donate blood if you are healthy. You can save a life.
- Blood products and transfusions can also transmit infections such as hepatitis, syphilis or HIV if contaminated with these infections.
- Blood and blood products are another "sensitive" subject especially with Jehovah's Witnesses who do not allow the receiving of blood products or transfusions by their followers. Talk about it with respect.
- Talk about the local blood transfusion services in the country.

Community story on blood transfusion policy

Athlone Hospital had a policy or guidelines of not to transfuse patients when their haemoglobin or blood concentration was 6gm % and above, which was seen as *"healthy"* in our circumstances, with the high HIV figures. The normal blood concentration level or haemoglobin in adults is 10-14 gm%.

Athlone Hospital rarely transfused pints of blood into patients, unless it was a life or death situation, such as in cases of ectopic pregnancies, where the baby is outside the womb or in the tubes. Blood transfusions were also given in road traffic accidents where there was massive bleeding or blood loss. Initially there was resistance to change, but with time the policy was taken on board when the hospital staff saw the good results of not transfusing patients routinely.

Routine blood transfusions were stopped in Athlone Hospital. We even had patients with blood concentrations of 5gm% that we did not transfuse and they never complicated or died.

Community story on a balanced diet and eating healthy

No AIDucation workshop is complete without discussing nutrition or food that must be eaten by people living with HIV infection or AIDS. The body's immune system ("soldiers") and blood concentration can be built up by a good, balanced diet.

Just as social workers are grossly under-utilised in the world of HIV infection and AIDS, so are dieticians and nutritionists. Invite them for your workshops. Remember that *"you are what you eat."*

LESSONS LEARNT

1. The decision of whether to give blood or not to a patient must be left to the doctors and nurses looking after the patients.

2. Blood transfusion policies must be revised or re-visited, especially with the advent of HIV infection and AIDS. Every blood transfusion given must be for a very strong reason

3. Remember blood saves lives. Be a blood donor and give blood.

4. AIDucation is about knowing and understanding the basic ways of HIV transmission – through sexual intercourse, pregnancy, breast feeding and through transfusion of contaminated blood products. Sharing or using blood contaminated needles, syringes and surgical instruments can be a source of HIV infection.

HIVT-F17: Universal precautions

ACTSAP

- Talk about infection control principles, health and safety in the workplace.

- Talk about sharps' containers and how to improvise where there are no such containers.

- Talk about biological or body waste and rubbish disposal in hospitals and in home based care.

TIPS

- Disposal or throwing away of needles and syringes in a proper way is very important whether it be at the hospital, clinic or at home, on home based care services. These containers with the needles and syringes should not be buried or thrown on the rubbish heap. The sharps' containers must be given to the hospital or the local council for incineration or burning.

- Discuss possibilities of needle stick pricks, injuries or accidents.

- Discuss actions to take when a healthcare worker is injured by a needle in the health facility or has been exposed to contaminated blood.

- Discuss what community members should do when pricked with a hospital needle at home during home based care. Washing of hands cannot be over emphasised.

- Mention the role of Post Exposure Prophylaxis (PEP). What is the policy about post-exposure prophylaxis or PEP in your country? Who is entitled to receiving PEP?

o In Botswana PEP was offered to rape victims and healthcare workers who had sustained needle stick injuries while on duty in the hospitals or clinics.

Community talking about health and safety

Athlone Hospital used this slide and script to write up its Infection Control Policy which was graded an "A+" by Ministry of Health in the early 1990s.

This slide led to the Ministry of health ordering yellow "sharps' containers" for the health facilities after Athlone Hospital had made an order for containers for "Health and Safety" at the workplace.

Blood and blood products should be treated with extreme care in waste management or disposal. Treat blood products as potentially infected and be careful of touching them with bare hands.

Community talking about rape and post-exposure prophylaxis (PEP)

Rape was treated as an emergency in Athlone Hospital. The Athlone Hospital staff working with the local police strived to see to it that the client or rape-victim was seen as soon as possible by the doctor on call. Police statements at the police station were done after the hospital visit.

When a woman was brought into the hospital with a reported sexual assault or rape, the hospital mobilised the medical officer on call, the pharmacy staff and the laboratory staff. Blood was collected, usually, within the hour after the rape. The rape victim was then started straight away on PEP. The follow-up, giving of the results and post-test counselling of the traumatised client was done by the social workers after two or three days, while the client was still taking the medication.

On a few occasions the PEP would be stopped, as the blood results, from the laboratory, showed that the woman who had been raped was already HIV positive before she was raped. She would be counselled and told her HIV status or position. The rape victim would be encouraged to contact her regular sexual partner(s) for HIV counselling and testing.

LESSONS LEARNT

1. Health and Safety programmes at the work place are very important programmes. Sadly these important programmes are grossly over looked.
2. Post exposure prophylaxis (PEP) medicines are given in many countries. Sadly many healthcare workers, rape victims or sexual assault victims do not know about these programmes in their countries.
3. Many police officers handling rape victims do not know about PEP.

HIVT-F18: Parent to child transmission of HIV

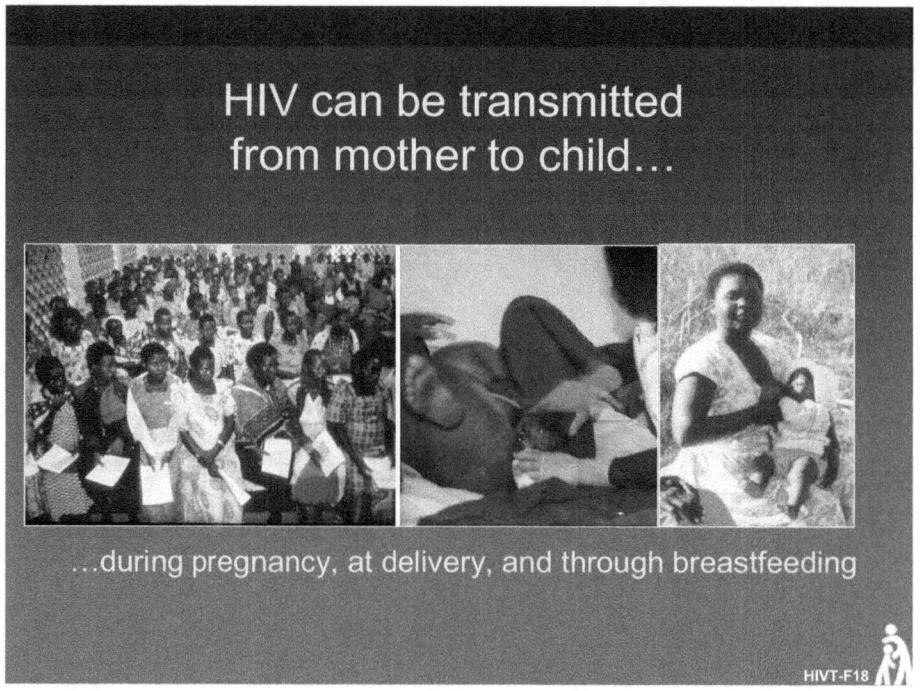

ACTSAP

- Talk about the routes of HIV transmission

- Talk about transmission of HIV infection during pregnancy, at child delivery or child birth and through breastfeeding

- Talk about the Prevention of the Mother To Child Transmission (PMTCT) of HIV infection programme.

TIPS

- o Let the women and mothers say as much as they can on pregnancy and HIV transmission. These three pictures will guide them.

- o Discuss what happens at the antenatal clinic and its importance

- o Discuss what happens at the Family Planning (FP) clinic

- o Discuss family planning and contraceptive methods

- o Talk about routine HIV testing before pregnancy

- o Dispel the myths and traditional beliefs surrounding HIV infection and pregnancy

- o Discuss what happens during the PMTCT programme and emphasise the role of breastfeeding in the PMTCT programme. Get participants to comment and debate on *"breast is best!"*

133

o Mothers at the Athlone Hospital antenatal clinic (ANC) sometimes spent the whole morning discussing these pictures on how HIV can be transmitted from the mother to the unborn child.

o Use these pictures to encourage carers or care-givers to always wear gloves when nursing patients who are HIV positive, especially where there is contact with body fluids and blood.

Community talking voluntary counselling and testing before pregnancy

Athlone Hospital had the earliest requests for voluntary counselling and testing (VCT) all because of the early Pictures in AIDucation awareness strategy in 1992. At one time there was a community outcry in early 1992 that Athlone Hospital was *"...alarmist"* and stating that hospital staff were saying that, *"...Pregnancy is an indirect test for HIV infection and AIDS. Dr Mapara told us so."*

From the early 1990s Athlone Hospital advised women to *"...test before pregnancy!"* Discussions were held about what an HIV positive test result meant and what were the risks of having an HIV infected baby. The facts were given and it was up to the women and their partners to decide on whether to have a baby or not to have a baby. Most of the babies born with HIV infection, by then never lived to see their fifth birthday. Pregnancy in some cases accelerated the development of AIDS in HIV infected women.

In the late 1990s the government introduced, *"Test before pregnancy"* through the Prevention of the Mother to Child Transmission (PMTCT) of HIV infection Programme.

Caesarean section operations in a world of HIV infection and AIDS

At Athlone Hospital, all our post-caesarean section (c/section) patients ate their food after 12 hours of having come from the operation theatre. We stopped waiting for 72 hours or for *"...bowel sounds heard..."* or *"...mother has passed wind (flatus)"* which we were taught at medical school in the 1980s. This action brought about better wound healing and bonding.

Simply put, mothers who delivered their babies by operation never *"starved"* for 48 to 72 hours afterwards. The mothers began to eat their food after 12 hours, in Athlone Hospital. Initially there was fear of burst abdomen, infections, operation complications and death. There was tension because of *"...another of Dr Mapara's experiments on our people!"* Those fears came to pass.

Healthcare workers who came from other hospitals marvelled at the Athlone Hospital style. Most of the hospitals were still starving mothers after the c/section operations. After three months of successful operations and eating after 12 hours from theatre, I asked the nurses if we could go back to the old style. They refused without hesitation and to this day the c/section operations are managed *"Mapara's way!"* Part of the Safe Motherhood Programme.

HIVT-F19: Influences on the risk of mother to child transmission of HIV

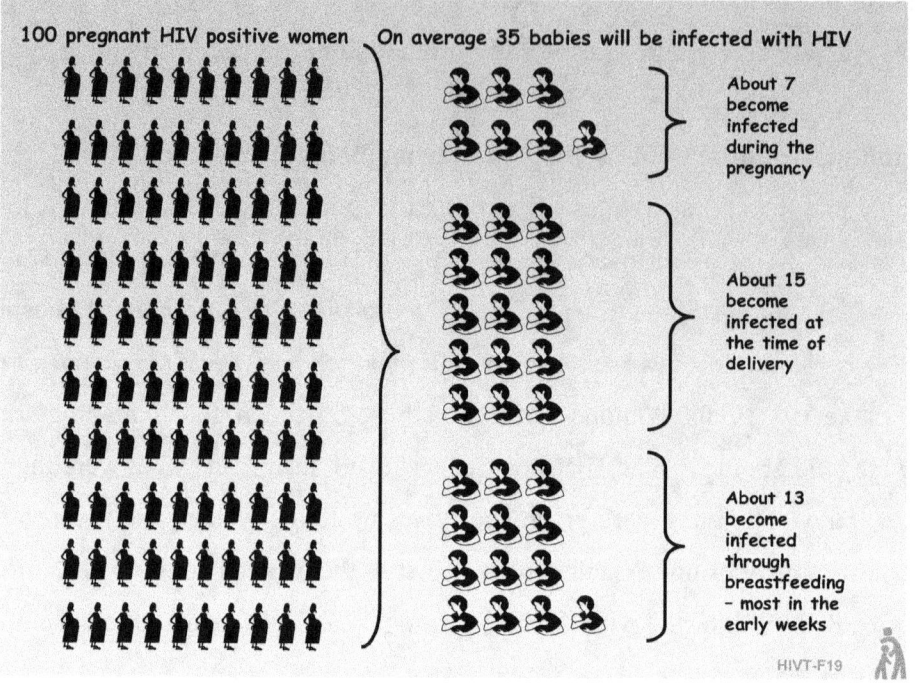

100 pregnant HIV positive women | On average 35 babies will be infected with HIV

About 7 become infected during the pregnancy

About 15 become infected at the time of delivery

About 13 become infected through breastfeeding – most in the early weeks

HIVT-F19

ACTSAP

- Talk about HIV positive pregnant mothers and risks of passing on HIV infection to the unborn babies
- Talk about the fact that less than half of the pregnant mothers who are HIV positive will transmit HIV infection to their babies
- Talk about HIV test before pregnancy and the registration on the PMTCT programme.

TIPS

- Discuss how HIV is transmitted from HIV positive pregnant mothers to the babies
- Allow the mothers to bring out all their concerns
- Never get tired of repeating the same message
- Remember that there is no such thing as a *"silly question or comment"* in AIDucation discussions.
- All the questions and comments are very relevant
- How are mothers delivered in places where there are no clinics? How are mothers delivered in the homes? Do the women or traditional birth attendants wear gloves?
- How are the biological wastes, the blood and the placenta disposed of or thrown away?

135

o Ask the participants, *"Do the traditional birth attendants or grandmothers wear gloves when conducting the deliveries in the homes? Are they protected?"*

o Ask the mothers, *"Why is that midwife or nurse in the middle picture wearing gloves?"*

Community talking traditional or home deliveries of babies

It is not uncommon to have grandmothers or elderly women help with delivering of babies at home when mothers go into labour. The women chase out all the young children and conduct the delivery in the bedroom. Do these women wear gloves? How do they cut the umbilical cord and with what? Where are the placenta and other waste products discarded or thrown away?

Another fact about the elderly women, mothers and grandmothers is that they like to go to the fields to cultivate or till the land with the traditional hoes. A few of the women end up with thorn pricks, cuts and bruises while out in the fields. What is the risk of HIV transmission if such women help in child birth or come in direct contact of HIV infected blood?

LESSONS LEARNT

1. There is no silly question or comment when it comes to talking about sexually transmitted infections, HIV infections or AIDS.

2. Remember that it was a "silly" comment that AIDS was an ***"American Ideology to Discourage Sex,"*** by the Lobatse students in 1992 that gave birth to the international teaching method of Pictures in AIDucation.

3. Everybody in this age and era should know about HIV infections and AIDS. All women must know issues around HIV infection, pregnancy and breastfeeding before becoming pregnant.

4. HIV infection and AIDS is about addressing gender issues.

HIVT-F20: The dilemma of breastfeeding and HIV transmission

ACTSAP

- Talk about the risk of HIV transmission through breastfeeding in a baby
- Talk about the risk of diarrhoea and malnutrition if baby not breastfed
- Talk about who decides on what is best for the baby.

TIPS

○ Should an HIV positive mother breastfeed or not?

○ What are the reasons for breastfeeding or not breastfeeding?

○ What are the options if the mother chooses not to breastfeed the baby for fear of passing on HIV infection through the breast milk? Is *"breast still best?"*

○ Are artificial feeds affordable? Is clean, boiled water available? Is the water stored properly and in what? Are the bottles properly washed?

Community talking PMTCT and *"...broadcasting"* HIV results

During the early days of the prevention of mother to child transmission (PMTCT) of HIV infection programmes in Africa, there was an issue of mothers choosing to have their newborn babies fed by other breastfeeding mothers or a sister or a relative. Does this still happen in the villages, rural areas or towns? What options are there?

Despite the PMTCT programme and the free tinned milk or supplementary feeds provided by the government, mothers feared being noticed, *"...carrying the blue tins"* of artificial milk from the health centres. The tinned milk *"...broadcasted a positive HIV result in the village"* said one mother who refused to join the PMTCT programme.

How can this stigma be reduced? What strategy can be used to distribute these supplementary feeds without *"...broadcasting"* to the community or unintentionally breaking the confidentiality and privacy agreed upon?

LESSONS LEARNT

1. Breastfeeding has to be discussed seriously before breastfeeding the newborn

2. Listen to the mothers with their concerns about *"...broadcasting"* their HIV status to the public, the neighbours, to immediate family members, mothers or mothers in law.

3. Confidentiality has to be respected in what ever we do.

   - How do you protect the mothers or women on the PMTCT programme from *"community stigmatisation"* as they register for the PMTCT programme?

HIVT-F21: Ways that HIV does not spread

HIV is *not* spread by...

- Mosquito bites
- Coughing
- Kissing
- Sharing cups or cutlery
- Hugging
- Shaking hands
- Using the toilet
- Using the telephone

HIVT-F21

ACTSAP

- Talk about how HIV infection is not spread, is not transmitted and is not acquired
- Talk about the body fluids that have high concentrations of HIV
- Talk about how HIV infection is transmitted
- Talk about HIV infection is transmitted, again.

TIPS

- Another set of pictures that are workshops on their own.
- Talk in the simplest of languages for everybody to understand that HIV infection is not transmitted in these ways shown in these pictures.
- Find out who disagrees with these pictures on how HIV infection is not spread and the reasons for disagreeing.
- Prepare to explain the questions around mosquito bites and why mosquitoes do not transmit HIV.
- Be ready for explaining *"deep kissing"* and *"light kissing"* in the spread of HIV infection
- Repeat the facts on how HIV infection is transmitted

- Stress that there are high concentrations of HIV in blood, semen, vaginal fluids and breast-milk.
- Ask participants for stories of stigma, discrimination or mistreatment of people living with HIV infection or AIDS.

Community talking stigma, discrimination and isolation

We have heard very sad stories of clients or people living with HIV infection and AIDS, who were humiliated, discriminated against or mistreated. They reported:

- *"I used a neighbour's dish to carry some vegetables in. Later I discovered that that very good dish was turned into a plate for the dogs, because I had used it!"*
- *"My aunt deliberately broke a glass that I had used to drink water in and threw it away. She even told her children to serve me water or food in special plastic plates and cups that were bought specifically for me when I visited them."*
- *"The staff-room tea cups and mugs that we used for drinking tea in were removed from the usual cupboard. All the teachers were coming with their own mugs, which they used, washed and put back in their bags. The key that used to be kept behind the door for the staff toilet was hidden from me. Everybody else knew where the key was, apart from me. Some teachers even feared to sit next to me. There was always an empty chair next to me!"* This was the experience of a teacher who was newly diagnosed HIV positive. He later asked the school authorities for a transfer to another school. The transfer was granted. The teacher did not reveal his HIV status in the new school.
- *"I make it a point to be the last one to use the showers at work. If I shower early, nobody will use the shower that I had used and they will all queue up for the other showers."* An HIV positive worker at one of the local factories sharing his *"...new life."*
- *"I had to get my child out of school, because the other parents were complaining and were threatening to remove their children from the school, after they heard that I was HIV positive. My child was healthy with no problems, but we still had to take him away. The headmaster understood my situation but there was nothing he could do!"* A mother living with HIV infection fighting for her child to remain in school. She lost the battle.
- *"Doc, it's nice to feel a human heart pounding on my chest again!"* A female client who was living with HIV infection. She had not been hugged for almost two years. In that AIDucation workshop, I hugged her and all the other participants followed my example. From zero hugs in two years to almost twenty hugs in one day.

- *"When my sister who is an educated nurse, comes to visit me, she never sits in the bath –tub when bathing and she never sits on the toilet seat. She squats in the bath-tub and she squats on the toilet seat! She fears to catch my disease!* A positive speaker stressing the need for healthcare workers to get AIDucated.

- *"Doctor, give these pictures to the other hospitals also. Those nurses mistreat us because they are very ignorant of these facts we have learnt. They wear masks when coming to give us our medicines!"* A disgruntled patient who was HIV positive and also had Kaposi's sarcoma.

- *"Ever since I left the hospital (about 4 weeks ago) you are the first one to touch me! No one has ever touched me or shaken my hand. They are all afraid of me because I have got AIDS. With your touch, I feel like a human being again."* These words were spoken by a lady who came for review at the out-patient department (OPD). I had casually put my arm on her shoulder as we talked, only for her to start crying. When I tried to remove my arm, thinking I had offended her, she told me not to remove it and explained why she was crying. I hugged her for almost two full minutes in front of all the patients and workers at the out-patient department. She sobbed, cried and laughed on my shoulders. We went off together, hand in hand, to the doctors' room for a cup of tea. She was my *"special guest"* on that day.

I was later told that the lady was not isolated anymore in the village. My hugging her in public had changed the village belief that *"...AIDS can be transmitted through touching and hugging a person with HIV infection!"* News travels fast. One report that I received about my hugging my client was, *"The AIDS doctor (the author) even kissed her on the lips!"*

LESSONS LEARNT

1. "Actions speak louder than words" said Jimmy Cliff. It is true.
2. You never know what small actions can bring about big changes and dispel myths.
3. Ignorance, stigma and discrimination are still very big issues out there. They need to be tackled by all of us.
4. I always hug clients living with HIV infection on the first day that I meet them or when they give their first public testimony on *"living with HIV infection"* in the AIDucation workshops. I have done this since 1985.

HIVT-F22: Prospects for an HIV vaccine

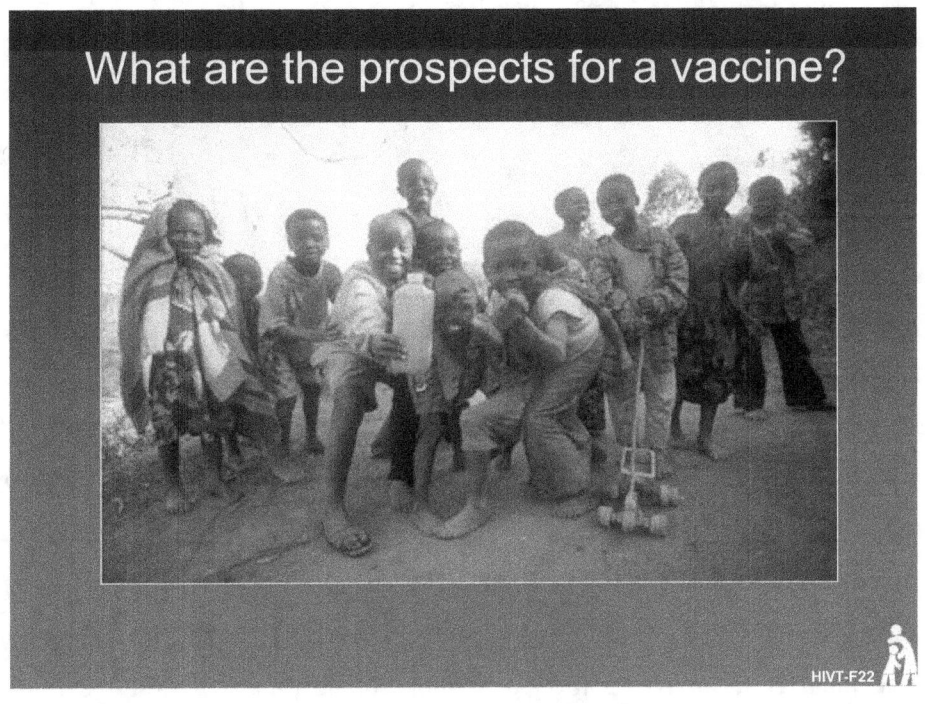

ACTSAP

- Talk about the chances of the scientists finding a vaccine for HIV

- Talk about vaccines and what vaccines do to the body, such as the BCG vaccine, DPT vaccine, measles vaccine and hepatitis vaccine

- Talk about the BCG vaccine and find out if anything has changed in terms of giving BCG to newborns, since HIV infection and AIDS came on the scene

- Talk about those scars on the left mid-arm or on the left shoulders of the AIDucation workshop participants. What is the cause of that scar?

TIPS

o I always ask, *"What are the chances for a vaccine?"*

o It is fascinating to see how many participants respond *"...never...not in our life-time...it will take a lot of years...the virus is too clever for us...with its changing skin there is no lock and key pattern...the virus will just one day die off and something else will start again!"*

o The participants respond in reference to the earlier pictures of the *"...changing...moving target...chameleon ...different from TB coat..."* pictures.

o Many participants stress the need for an aggressive HIV infection and AIDS awareness campaign as *"...money is being wasted looking for a vaccine..."* while many people are being infected out of lack of basic life saving knowledge.

o The enlightened discussion and debate is usually one of my markers that the message has got home, that learning has taken place.

o Adult learning needs patience.

o The only *"vaccine"* we have today is Pictures in AIDucation, Pictures in AIDucation and more Pictures in AIDucation.

Community talking about "Sex Education"

This picture of the children playing somehow always stimulates the discussion on sex education. What is sex education? When do we start talking sex and relationships to our children? When do we start imparting life saving skills? Who is responsible for initiating or starting dialogue on sex education? Is it the parents or relatives at home? Is it the teachers at school or is it the faith ministers at church or the imams at the mosques? Whose responsibility is it to AIDucate the young ones?

One headmaster in an AIDucation workshop for headmasters said, *"Children of nowadays should start being taught about sex and relationships by the time they are nine or ten years old. After all some of them have their own babies at the age of twelve or fourteen, which was unheard of in our times! If we do not want AIDS to wipe out these children, we should have started talking all these things (sexually transmitted infections) to them yesterday."*

Some teachers and headmasters laughed at this comment and suggestion. *"This is no laughing matter!"* he added in a very stern headmaster's voice as he sat down. There was a harsh from the colleagues. Food for thought!

LESSONS LEARNT

1. Parents are silent on sex matters. Are you, your school and Parents Teachers Association (PTA) doing enough in terms of sex education and AIDucation?

2. Schools should start serious sex education and AIDucation as early as possible.

3. Church silence, school silence, work place silence and community silence help to spread sexually transmitted infections, HIV infection and AIDS. Silence is a catalyst to active transmission of HIV infection.

HIVT-F23: Treatment for HIV infection

ACTSAP

- Talk about no cure to date for HIV infection or for AIDS

- Talk briefly about antiretroviral therapy (ART) or anti-HIV drugs

- Talk about the national criteria being used to start or commence a client or person living with HIV infection or AIDS on treatment.

TIPS

- There are anti-HIV drugs that can improve the quality of life for people living with HIV infection or AIDS. Mention the classes or groups of drugs and what is special about some of them in terms of when to drink them or how to drink them or how to store them

- For many participants, treatment, ART is like a dream. It is out of reach. Is this true?

- Emphasise that not all clients who test HIV positive should start treatment immediately. There is a protocol or treatment criteria that is followed.

- The developing countries are still struggling to put all their people living with HIV infection and AIDS on treatment.

- Participants should give examples of what is happening in their districts about treatment programmes and the PMTCT programmes. What are the challenges?

Community talking "…*die a little bit more*" to qualify for HIV infection treatment

"Doctor, are you telling us that a patient who has HIV infection has to die a little bit more for him or her to qualify for the AIDS drugs?" This was a question asked by a participant in an AIDucation workshop as we talked about the reduction in CD4 cell counts ("soldiers") in the body, the increased viral load or concentration or volume or amount of the virus in the body and the treatment criteria.

How does one answer such a genuine question? I gave the participant my answer. What answer would you give the participant on *"…dying a little bit more to qualify for treatment?"*

Community talking from experience… *"Thank you for teaching me about me."*

After three consecutive Saturdays with the youths on an AIDucation course, we wound up the course with an evaluation on paper and chatting about the course. We went round the horse-shoe sitting arrangement. All the fourteen participants, youths, gave a positive feedback and wished that, *"AIDucation could be taught in the schools. We do not have sex education in the schools."*

One 17 years old teenager stood up, when it came to his turn to comment about the three Saturdays of AIDucation. He said, *"Doc, thank you for teaching me about me!"* I was a bit confused with this statement. As I was gathering my thoughts, the young man put his hand into his right pocket of his trousers and brought out the same container of Triomune (Nevirapine), seen in the picture above. You should have seen the shocked and surprised expressions of the other participants. For three Saturdays we had a friend with HIV infection in our midst and we did not know it.

As usual, according to my tradition from Zambia, I walked over and hugged the young man. I thanked him for his courage of revealing his HIV status to us, who were literally strangers. The others all came and hugged him to. I asked him if he would mind talking to us about his life as a person living with HIV infection. He did not mind. For thirty minutes he spoke about his young life. For thirty minutes he answered questions from all of us. For thirty minutes he made HIV infection visible. He had given a human face to our three Saturdays of AIDucation.

LESSONS LEARNT

1. The grassroots folks or community members might understand doctors and nurses differently in interpreting scientific facts. Do not assume.

2. Be patient in your discussions. We do not all understand things the same way.

HIVT-F24: A continuum of care

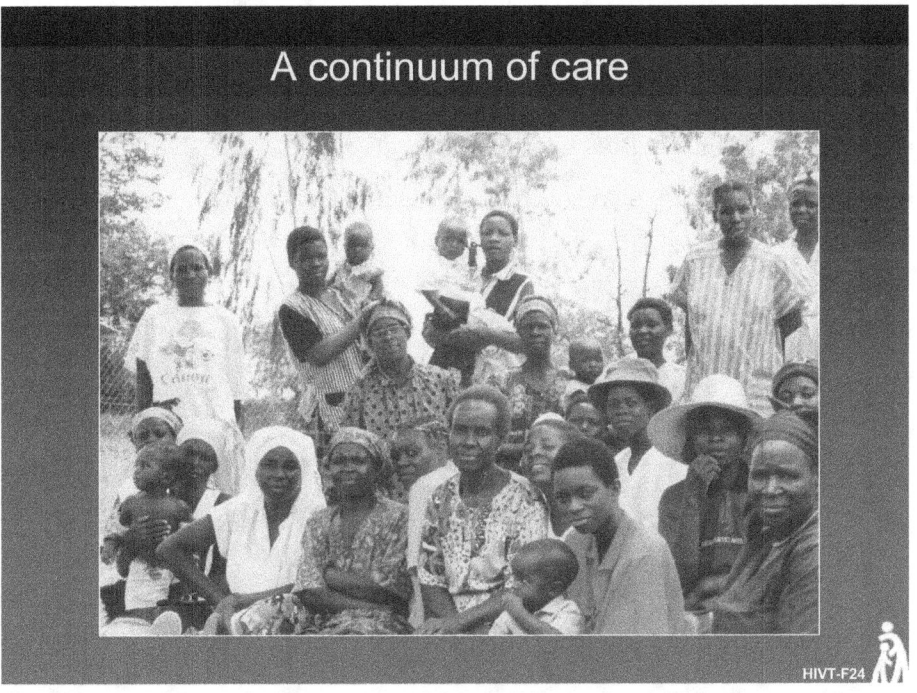

A continuum of care

"It takes a village to raise a child."

African saying

ACTSAP

- Talk about this picture representing the AIDucation workshop participants
- Talk about what makes us different from these folks in the picture
- Talk about what makes us similar to these folks.

TIPS

o This picture is used to *"jump start"* community members into action. These are ordinary village folks who are actively engaged in HIV infection and AIDS activities.

o The day these community members can give talks and facilitate discussions using the AIDucation pictures and videos, then you know that your HIV infection and AIDS awareness raising programme has succeeded.

o If these folks cannot teach or talk on HIV infection and AIDS in the village then we are in a lot of trouble. he future is bleak.

o If HIV infection and AIDS are still treated as health issues, with healthcare workers alone giving talks, then we still have many more of our brothers and sisters to bury before their time. AIDS is a developmental problem and not a health problem only.

Some AIDucation participants (country) who have viewed these pictures over the twenty years of Botswana's AIDucation include:

A.   Angola, Australia and America

B.   Barbados, Belgium, Botswana and Britain

C.   Canada, Caribbean Islands, Chad, China and Cuba

D.   Denmark and Democratic Republic of Congo (DRC)

E.   Ecuador and Egypt

F.   France

G.   Ghana and Guinea Bissau

H.   Haiti and Holland

I.   Ireland, Italy, Iran and Ivory Coast

J.   Jamaica

K   Kenya

L.   Lesotho

M.   Malawi, Mauritius and Mozambique

N.   Namibia and Nigeria

P.   Philipines and Poland

R.   Russia and Rwanda

S.   Saudi Arabia, Senegal, Somalia, South Africa, Spain, Sudan and Swaziland

T.   Tanzania and Turkey

U.   Uganda

Z.   Zambia and Zimbabwe.

AIDUCATION

Questions on HIV infection and AIDS should be asked freely. Do not be shy or embarrassed. We all have the right to question on the facts of life and to receive life saving information.

Red ribbon worn on the left side of the chest shows that you care for and support people living with HIV infection and AIDS in the community.

PART THREE

Athlone Hospital Health Resource Centre services

- o Counselling

- o Information dissemination

- o AIDucation

- o Facilitating at workshops

- o Assisting research and project students

- o Help with adjustment to hospitalisation

- o HIV testing

- o Networking with other agencies

- o Training of trainers

- o Telephone help-line

- o Support elective attachments

- o Data collection

- o Evaluation and monitoring

- o Sign-posting

- o Hosting local and international visitors

- o Helping in setting up other health resource centres in Botswana.

10. HEALTH RESOURCE CENTRES IN BOTSWANA

"Until the lion has his own story-teller, the hunter will always have the best part of the story."

African saying

The first health resource centre in Botswana

The Ministry of Health and the AIDS/STD Unit had turned down the Project Proposal for setting up the Athlone Hospital Health Resource Centre (AHRC) in Lobatse, after the 1997 AIDucation "National Tour of Hope." This did not stop the *"...too ambitious"* plans of Athlone Hospital. The vision of AHRC, pronounced "Ark" was going to be realised through faith and perseverance. Noah in the Bible did not have it easy when building the Ark. He was mocked and ridiculed. Nonetheless Noah remained focussed and he persisted until the ark was built, with God on his side. This old Bible story of the "floods (equated to HIV infection and AIDS)" was Athlone Hospital's inspiration. Amen.

The Athlone Team had only one vision, to build the AHRC. With God on our side, through the Athlone Spiritual Committee and with financial help from the Athlone Hospital Advisory Committee, failure was not an option. The Athlone team turned to its faithful village members through the Hospital Advisory Committee (HAC), chaired by Mrs Mbulawa, the head teacher of Itireleng Secondary school and the Patron, Mr Goolam Asmal, a very successful businessman. The "Athlone Way" never failed us. The Project Proposal for the health resource centre was presented to the Hospital Advisory Committee who promised to make Athlone Hospital's vision a reality.

Our prayers were answered. With support and fund-raising by the local Lobatse community, spear-headed by the Hospital Advisory Committee, the first health resource centre in Botswana was born at Athlone Hospital, Lobatse, on the 30th November 1999. The Athlone Health Resource Centre was officially opened on 30th November 1999 by Mr Goolam Asmal, the Patron. The AHRC has stood firm and has played its national role in the Botswana HIV infection and AIDS epidemics.

It must be emphasised, repeated and stressed that the Athlone Hospital Health Resource Centre **"The AHRC" was built from the money raised by the community members of Lobatse**. There was no financial support or assistance from the Ministry of Health or the AIDS/STD Unit as it was not seen as a viable project. The AHRC was built on the rock solid foundation of Pictures in AIDucation. The AHRC was built through faith.

149

The vision had finally become reality. The rest is history. Now talk about the other health resource centres modelled around the *"Mother Model"* in Lobatse, at Athlone Hospital.

Athlone Hospital Health Resource Centre Profile

Location

Athlone Health Resource Centre (AHRC) is located behind the hospital staff car park and opposite the Pharmacy Department.

Background

The Health Resource Centre was officially opened on the 30th November 1999.

The centre was set up after the Athlone AIDS Awareness Project and the Social Work Department realised a need for a client to meet all his/her needs under one roof.

This was done by integrating the services offered by the Athlone AIDS Awareness Programme and the Social Work Department.

Philosophy

The Health Resource Centre and Social Work Department are proactive in advocating for patients and their families. We subscribe to the Ministry of Health's emphasis on disease prevention, health promotion, curative and rehabilitation services.

Capacity

Two full-time nurse counsellors and three social workers work in the centre on full time basis. A medical doctor (originally Dr Mapara) is called in when needed.

Goal

Provide information, education and counselling services on different types of health and social issues. Some of the issues addressed are diabetes, HIV infection, AIDS, cancer, rape, suicide, family problems, domestic violence etc.

Main activities

- Counselling
- Information, education and communication
- Referrals / Sign-posting.

Services provided

1. Counselling on health and social matters.
2. Information, education and communication on health and social issues with emphasis on sexually transmitted infections (STI), in particular HIV infection and AIDS as they are a great threat to our community.

3. Facilitation of workshops on behalf of other organisations e.g. schools, non-governmental organisations, government departments, community and multi-sectoral AIDS committees.

4. Assisting students from various schools with research projects.

5. Pre and post test counselling for HIV infection and AIDS is offered.

6. On-going or supportive counselling for both HIV positive and HIV negative clients.

7. Give information on the importance of drug treatment and adherence.

8. Help with the adjustment to hospitalisation.

9. Provide or act as a link between the hospital and the community as well as other organisations. Networking.

10. Training of Trainers (TOT) in HIV infection and AIDS education (AIDucation).

11. Telephone helpline. On-going counselling or information sharing by telephone.

12. Assist and supervise Institute of Development Management (IDM) and University of Botswana (UB) Social Work students on internship.

13. Collect information on services provided by different organisations outside the hospital and refer the clients appropriately. Sign-posting.

Target Group

Athlone Hospital assists patients that come to the centre for assistance. These include health workers and the general public.

People are treated equally regardless of their ethnic, political, nationality, socio-economic status, background or gender.

Source: AHRC leaflet designed by M.M.Mothlake, Chairman Athlone Hospital, AIDSAwareness Project, 2000

The Botswana 1990 *"best practice"* Athlone Hospital AIDS Awareness Programme and the Botswana 1999 *"best practice"* Athlone Health Resource Centre owe their documented successes to the leadership of the Hospital Advisory Committee, the Athlone Hospital Management Team and the faithful community of Lobatse. The leadership was approached twice for assistance. The leadership twice believed and twice generously supported the Athlone Hospital AIDucation team. The leadership got it right twice, to initiate and pioneer local projects that became national *"best practice"* programmes.

The Botswana health resource centres would play a major role in the provision of anti-AIDS drugs or antiretroviral therapy. Many international organisations have come into Botswana to give a helping hand in providing anti-HIV drugs or treatment for people living with HIV infection and AIDS, but did not know the history of the resource centres. The roots are in Lobatse.

This is living testimony that African communities talking sex, AIDS and pictures in Lobatse had made history. Pula (Let it rain)!

Replication of Athlone Hospital Health Resource Centre

In 2001, the Botswana government in partnership with its many international partners began to replicate the Athlone Hospital *"Mother Model"* Health Resource Centre nation wide, in the twenty-four health districts. Maun General Hospital was the second health resource centre to go up in October 2001. The dream was being realised. Athlone Hospital would lead and others would follow.

Athlone Hospital was called upon by the Ministry of Health, Botswana, to write up the official opening speech for the second centre that was to open at Maun General Hospital. The speech writing for the official opening of the Maun General Hospital Health Resource Centre was delegated to Athlone Hospital as *"...You are the ones who know what a health resource centre is!"* Take note, that at that time in 2001, there was only one health resource centre in Botswana. Where was it? At Athlone Hospital, Lobatse, the home of the Athlone AIDS Awareness Project and Pictures in AIDucation intervention strategy.

The Maun speech was written and delivered within the hour of the request, using points from "Phaks" Mmothlake's leaflet on the Athlone Health Resource Centre.

Almost like the Cinderella story. What was once a *"thorn in the flesh"* in 1990 had become the *"corner-stone"* for the Botswana AIDS programme in the year 2000 AD. This is testimony to the fact that **African Communities Talking Sex, AIDS and Pictures** can develop local, national and international HIV infection and AIDS Programmes. Who better than the communities grossly affected and living with the impact of HIV infection and AIDS to teach others on prevention, care and support initiatives? There is no excuse for Africa not to lead and excel.

It is a fact that HIV infection and AIDS is in the village and the solution to addressing HIV infection and AIDS is in the village with the people who live with AIDS every single day. The Livingstone, Zambia and Lobatse, Botswana programmes are testimony to this fact.

In July 2002, at the international conference on HIV infection and AIDS held in Barcelona, Spain, the Botswana Government and its many partners spoke about its *"successful"* projects, that included the Health Resource Centres in Botswana, but with one exception - Athlone Hospital Resource Centre did not feature anywhere in their documentation or discussion. You can imagine the feelings and the emotions of the Athlone team and the community of Lobatse. We will not go into the details, but just to say that *"ouch"*, it hurt! For the first time in twelve years, there was *"mistrust"* in the Athlone team. We had always looked after each other, until "Barcelona 2000". Some *"A Team"* members believed that *"...the doctor (Dr Mapara) has betrayed us and sold us to the Americans!"*

Meanwhile other HIV infection and AIDS prevention, care and support programmes that government supported, that had already been established such as the Botswana Christian AIDS Intervention Programme (BOCAIP), Botswana Network of People Living with HIV infection and AIDS (BONEPWA) and The Coping Centre for People living with HIV infection and AIDS (COCEPWA) were all documented and mentioned at "Barcelona 2002". These are organisations that were born years after Athlone Hospital AIDS Awareness Project and with a *"...little help"* from the very friendly, non-discriminating Athlone Hospital AIDS Awareness team.

The Botswana "Barcelona 2002" team internationally forgot to mention Athlone Hospital with the original *"Mother Model"* Health Resource Centre that was born two years before any other health resource centre in Botswana and was the trend-setter in the district hospitals.

To add salt to the wound, the Botswana "Barcelona 2002" team, locally remembered, in the month of August 2002, to ask Athlone Hospital to facilitate at a national workshop on *"Athlone Health Resource Centre's Experiences"* for district and referral hospital management teams (Chief Medical Officers, Matrons and Administrators) in Gaborone. The Athlone Hospital team gladly facilitated, doing what it did best, on the understanding that Athlone Hospital AIDS Awareness Programme would receive support, which was long overdue, from the organisers of this national conference. Did the support come as per agreement? No, sadly and unfortunately, the support that was agreed on never came. In the civil service we do the job and complain later. Serving God given lives is more important than man's worldly material contracts.

The truth of the matter was that the workshop organisers had heard that Dr Edwin Mapara, the pioneer of Athlone Hospital's successful AIDS awareness projects, was leaving for the United Kingdom, after twelve years of active involvement in almost all of Botswana's HIV infection and AIDS intervention strategies in Botswana. *"Athlone Health Resource Centre's Experiences"* Workshop was his last official assignment, as the Chief Medical Officer of Athlone Hospital and the national AIDucator. It was time to go and challenge the North or the developed countries.

On 16th August 2002 Dr Edwin Mavunika Mapara officially bowed off the Botswana stage. He said good-bye to Botswana as he began to prepare for a **self-sponsored** postgraduate course at the London School of Hygiene and Tropical Medicine, University of London, in the United Kingdom. For the records it was not funded or sponsorship by the Botswana government or *"The Americans"*, it was a self-sponsored Master of Science in Infectious Diseases postgraduate degree programme.

153

Monitoring and evaluation of HIV infection and AIDS programmes

Coincidentally, three days later, an independent team of five consultants conducted the terminal evaluation of the Programme Support Document (PSD), 1997 – 2002. The evaluation was conducted between 19th August and 18th November 2002. The Report of the terminal evaluation was printed on 10th December 2002. Athlone Hospital AIDS Awareness Programme featured in the report. Some extracts from the report that touch or mention Athlone Hospital are:

a.) Policy Development

√ The Athlone Hospital had formed an AIDS committee in line with the requirements of the PSD

b.) Capacity Building

√ A Health Resource Centre had been established within Athlone Hospital for training, service delivery and the follow up of clients. The Centre fulfils four main functions;

o Education and counselling of clients and families

o Serves as a resource centre and training centre

o Serves as a family support centre

o Serves as a continuum of care centre.

The Athlone Hospital in Lobatse with support from the District Multi-sectoral AIDS Committee has trained 120 HIV/AIDS trainers to raise the capacity of the institution for providing the continuum of care to patients on antiretroviral therapy who inevitably always came back to Athlone for management, care and support as soon as they were released from the antiretroviral therapy centre in Gaborone.

c.) Constraints and implementation gaps

√ Inadequate technical assistance and support has been provided to the staff of the Health Resource Centre as it is assumed that they are self-sufficient, capable and informed. Their own learning needs, as well as their needs for counselling and coping with the challenges in their work, has not been assessed and targeted with efficient interventions.

√ Inadequate exposure of the staff in the Health Resource Centre to educational and other staff development opportunities available in the region and internationally.

d.) Recommendations

√ The newly established AIDS information and counselling services including the Health Resource Centre should be assessed to identify priorities and areas to be strengthened. Similarly best practice experiences should be replicated for the expansion of the response.

Under **"Emerging best practice and interventions"** the document states:
The five years of Programme Support Document program implementation has brought it some best practice experiences and lessons learned that can be shared with countries elsewhere and be used to scale up selected program areas. A selection of what is considered best practice is described below as "targeted" and "emergent" as the program was evolving.

Emergent:

√ The establishment of AIDS Information and Counselling Centres and Health Resource Centres has been stimulated by the PSD. This innovation is currently being replicated in public and private institutions, as well as in the formal and informal sectors.

A village public health programme finally given its rightful status

Athlone Hospital, the Hospital Advisory Committee with the Lobatse community had made history that both local and foreign consultants would learn from for many years to come, so long as HIV infection and AIDS were still with us. Lobatse had climbed and conquered the mountain. Vision with action had become a reality. The 1990 *"...too ambitious and not possible...stubborn..."* Athlone AIDS Awareness Programme was elevated to an international AIDucation programme.

Oh what sweet music to the ears. *"Congratulations Lobatse! Congratulations Athlone Hospital!"* Let us hear it one more time for the unsung heroes of Lobatse village in Botswana that,

"The establishment of AIDS Information and Counselling Centres and Health Resource Centres has been stimulated by the PSD. This innovation is currently being replicated in public and private institutions, as well as in the formal and informal sectors

(PSD Report, published on 10th December 2002). "

AIDUCATION

Sexual intercourse is the main way of HIV transmission in Africa. Silence about sexual intercourse, sexuality and sexual relationships fuels the spread of HIV infection.

Transmission of HIV infection is through sexual intercourse and transfusion of unscreened or HIV contaminated blood. HIV can also be transmitted during pregnancy, at child birth, through breast-feeding, through use of contaminated needles, syringes and surgical equipment.

PART 4

AIDucation "D" issues on antiretroviral therapy (ART)

- o Drugs and community dialogue

- o Doses and number of tablets

- o Drinking medicine at specified times

- o Drinking medicine alone and not sharing with others

- o Drug side-effects to be anticipated

- o Drug side-effects and response

- o Duration or length of treatment

- o Drug resistance or reduced power

- o Diseases to be mentioned to the doctor or the nurse

- o Drink (Alcohol or beer) and traditional medicines

- o Double infection of HIV infection and tuberculosis

- o *"Dangerous"* or *"poisonous"* drugs

- o Drugs and death

- o Drugs and the *"Lazarus effect"*
- o Drugs and AIDucators.

Dr Edwin Mavunika Mapara

11. BOTSWANA'S ANTIRETROVIRAL THERAPY PROGRAMME

"You have to look after wealth, but knowledge looks after you."

African saying

Athlone Hospital's second national assignment

Botswana took a very bold step to start providing antiretroviral therapy (ART) to its people living with HIV infection and AIDS. President Festus Mogae of Botswana scored 100% on this bold decision in 2001. It was the right decision. With the world watching Botswana on its *"...too ambitious"* programme, Athlone Hospital was preparing to do what it had been yearning to do for the last decade, to put into place a Public Health School on AIDucation and a *"blue-print"* for a health resource centre. It was now or never. Providing antiretroviral therapy to Botswana called for courage, drive, determination, dedication, decentralisation and delegation.

While Dr Edwin Mapara was based in Gaborone, with the National Antiretroviral Therapy (ART) Project Team, from June 2001 to August 2001, Athlone Hospital was planning one step ahead. Athlone Hospital was determined to see the ART Project in Botswana become a reality. Athlone Hospital AIDS Awareness team had read about the Brazilian ART Programme and that had convinced the team that if there was a country in Africa to do it, Botswana could with its economic advantage. Despite other short-comings especially with manpower, we could only know if we tried. Risks had to be taken. This was one hell of a risk and somehow the Athlone team was very confident we would achieve our aims.

There was a high likelihood, from the grapevine, that the author, Dr Mapara, would be one of the team members that might be appointed to run the first Botswana National ART Programme. The programme would be fully funded by the Botswana government and its international partners. When the appointment came, Dr Mapara began mobilising the various partners and organisations that were involved in HIV infection and AIDS prevention, care and support activities that Athlone Hospital had worked with in the past. These were the Botswana Network of people living with HIV infection and AIDS (BONEPWA), Botswana Christian AIDS Intervention Programme (BOCAIP), Total Community Mobilisation (TCM), The Tebelopele Voluntary Counselling and Testing (VCT) centres, Teachers in the Ministry of Education and finally healthcare workers from the selected four initial ART sites, namely, Gaborone, Francistown, Serowe and Maun.

Dr Mapara kept the team leaders of these organisations posted and told them to be prepared and to be ready for a short notice call up for AIDucation workshops at Athlone Hospital, in Lobatse.

Why Lobatse? The team in Lobatse was ready for action and national duty. The Athlone team had ten years of experience of AIDucation, training of trainers (TOT) and helping to develop HIV infection and AIDS control programmes across Botswana. Athlone had the capacity and the know how.

The plan was to start sensitising the grassroots folks in the villages much earlier, before the arrival of the anti-HIV drugs in the village, if we were to succeed in this mammoth task or *"...experimenting with our people..."* as some people thought. The feasibility study, of June 2001 to August 2001, showed that Botswana was really going to start from a point of weakness, in terms of resources, apart from the substantial funds and a dedicated *"head-hunted"* team. The June to August 2001 assignment did not paint a pretty picture at all. Botswana had gross problems or rather major challenges to meet.

As Mike Lipkin, the South African motivational speaker would say, *"Yeeesssss! Challenges are meant to be overcome!"* The challenges that Botswana had were massive, but they could be overcome with time, dedication and faith. The challenges were:

- **Centralisation of the HIV infection and AIDS Programmes**

   This was a major issue. The HIV infection and AIDS Programmes were too centralised and based in the capital city, Gaborone. This had more of disadvantages than advantages. For a successful distribution of the anti-HIV drugs, there was need for decentralisation and power to be handed to the various district hospitals and AIDS awareness community programmes. Many districts had the potential to manage with some support from the National AIDS Coordinating Agency (NACA). It will be very unfair not to mention Ms Monica Tselayakgosi for her support when Athlone Hospital approached her, at all times, even at the eleventh hour.

- **Critical manpower shortages**

   Medical doctors, nurses, paramedics, social workers, counsellors, pharmacists, laboratory personnel, administrative officers, people living with HIV infection and AIDS as buddies or adherence counsellors, media advocates and community hands for home based care needed to be trained, found or recruited.

- **Poor physical infrastructure and lack of office spaces**

   Hospitals, clinics, office space, counselling space, health resource centres and safe drug storage space had to be built, created or simply found. The HIV infection and AIDS epidemics were calling for new physical infrastructure and resources.

- **Lack of laboratory capacity, equipment and reagents**

   Botswana needed new laboratories, upgrading of existing ones, purchasing of new testing equipment, assorted reagents and safer methods of working with blood samples. Gaborone and Francistown alone could not cope. Services had to be out-sourced.

- **Lack of comprehensive pharmaceutical logistics**

  Systems had to be re-visited in terms of ordering drugs, procurement, transportation, storage, refrigeration and distribution. Pharmacists, who were a rare commodity, were very essential for the implementation of the anti-HIV drugs programme. Sadly the pharmacists were in short supply and pharmacy technicians had to undergo a lot of vigorous training for the work still to come as part of the coping mechanism.

- **Insufficient social services, counselling and emotional support services**

  Social services had not been very important in HIV infection and AIDS management, until now. The HIV infection and AIDS epidemics had exposed Botswana's shortfalls. Social workers were finally important in running AIDS Programmes, by virtue of their training. They are more of counsellors than doctors and nurses. They do not just *"...pakisa dijo hela (pack food only)"* or hand out rations, as they are usually abused. Social workers are key players in HIV infection and AIDS control programmes. Africa delayed in learning this fact.

  Colleagues who went to Brazil in 2002 to see how the Brazilians were managing their HIV infection and AIDS crisis came back impressed and shocked. One colleague said, *"Edwin you were right. Social workers are heading AIDS Programmes in Brazil and have physicians working under them in a multi-disciplinary team."* How possible is this in Africa?

- **Inadequate HIV infection and AIDS information, education and communication (IEC)**

  The information and education programmes could have been better managed with Botswana's wide mass media communications network. This is where Athlone Hospital would have led with the Public Health School in AIDucation, AIDucating colleagues, who would equally AIDucate their various communities. Not blowing our (Athlone Hospital) trumpet, but simply stating a fact, Athlone Hospital in terms of AIDucation was second to none in the early and late 1990s. AIDucators were born in Athlone Hospital.

- **Irregular monitoring and evaluation of HIV infection and AIDS Programmes**

  Generally the national monitoring and evaluations of *"...best practices"* was far and wide. The local community programmes have to be reviewed constantly, at least every six months or even less, especially in the initial stages to replicate what is replicable and to remove what is removable, not working. Consultation with the local programmes is very important. Having faith in the active local (Botswana) programmes is equally important.

- **Lack of computer equipment (hardware and software)**

  These had to be put in place. Healthcare workers had to be trained in the hundreds as an emergency. For many of us, computers were not part of our daily lives. The internet, surfing the web, online discussions and emails were foreign, especially with the older generation of officers. Computers are very important for the management and follow-up of clients on anti-HIV drugs, as we respect confidentiality.

The young generations coming out of African schools, colleges and universities understand computers and information technology (IT) very much. Give the local young computer geniuses a chance before you call in the foreign IT consultants, who your young ones might end up teaching, as has happened in many other programmes. You can ask me.

- **Lack of support for local *"best practice"* AIDS Awareness and control programmes**

  Suffice to say that Botswana lost many opportunities that would have made a big difference, had it supported its own people and programmes more in the early years of the HIV infection and AIDS epidemics. Good documented examples are the Athlone AIDS Awareness Programme (AAAP) of 1990, Athlone Hospital's "Pictures in HIV/AIDS education (AIDucation)" initiative of 1992 and Athlone Health Resource Centre (AHRC) of 1999, as stated by a few, genuine, foreign consultants.

- **Lack of belief in Pictures in AIDucation**

  Despite Pictures in AIDucation being a cheap, cost-effective way of raising awareness on HIV infection and AIDS it was still, mostly, a Lobatse programme. Yet we know that, *"...A picture is worth a thousand words"* and *"seeing is very different from being told."* AIDucation will become an international intervention strategy. Keep an ear to the ground.

Called to perform

The beauty of implementing the Botswana anti-HIV drugs programme or antiretroviral therapy programme, in 2001, was that everybody was being called upon to do what they had been trained to do as doctors, nurses, social workers, counsellors, pharmacists, laboratory technicians, computer personnel, researchers, administrators, health promoters and teachers.

Each cadre was essential and played a major part in meeting these challenges. The doctors and nurses could not cope anymore and were being forced to *"let go"* and de-medicalise HIV infection and AIDS, finally. In some cases the doctors and nurses had been stumbling blocks. The healthcare workers were simply overwhelmed and quite a number were burnt-out. More hands were needed and there were thousands of free hands in the villages, waiting to be called into action after empowerment through AIDucation.

Botswana did not have the ideal *"enabling factors"* to run such a national programme, but she had no option. It was either she tried or she died. I could not picture the hundreds of people dying without a fight. I had waited too long for this moment and opportunity. I would not let this President Festus Mogae given chance slip by. The journey had been long and painful, but we were almost there. We had lost and buried too many of our brothers, sisters, mothers, fathers, uncles, aunts, friends and children to HIV infection and AIDS, the trend had to be stopped or slowed down.

We had no choice and for me, two sentences gave me hope on the day that the Antiretroviral Therapy Project Team met the President of Botswana, His Excellency President Festus Mogae and the Honourable Minister of Health, Mrs Joy Phumaphi in June 2001. The President told us that, *"...Failure is not an option."* The instruction was loud and clear. *"Money must not be an issue,"* said the Minister of Health who also added, *"...you have been chosen for this national project, because of your track records, at your various stations."* Those were very inspiring and motivating words. The Athlone Hospital *"...stubbornness"* had finally paid off.

The 1990 Athlone spirit was rekindled immediately. Deep down I knew that I was long ready and that we would make a difference. The Lobatse community was ready. Athlone Hospital was ready and the Athlone team was ready for the national assignment.

Of the close to three hundred thousand (300,000) people living with HIV infection and AIDS in Botswana in the year 2000, the study and investigations that we had conducted, had shown that close to 100, 000 people living with HIV infection and AIDS needed to be put on treatment. The village folks had to be mobilised to help the infected and affected. Time was not on our side, but that was no reason for failure.

The "D" issues on antiretroviral therapy

The village or town folks had to know what government was planning to do and what these anti-HIV drugs, *"...ART...ARVs..."* were and what was so special about them. We needed the community support, trust and cooperation for the success of the project. That could only come through discussions, initiated by Pictures in AIDucation. These drugs were not like any other drugs in terms of the *"...D..."* issues listed and had to be discussed for better understanding:

- **Dialogue** on drugs through PICTURES in AIDucation
- **Doses** or NUMBER of tablets to be taken
- **Drinking** them at the specified TIMES, before or after meals and reasons given
- **Drinking** them alone and NOT SHARING them with other family members who might be living with HIV infection or AIDS in the same house or house-hold
- **Drug side-effects** to be ANTICIPATED in some cases

- **Drug side-effects** and how to RESPOND to these effects, including not to stop taking the treatment until the patient is seen by the doctor or nurse who would advise on what to do next.

- **Duration** of treatment or ART being for LIFE OR FOREVER. Recall, *"...stepping on the head of a snake"* and *"...treatment is like a marriage, but with no room for divorce."*

- **Drug resistance** and meaning. Recall the CHANGING nature of HIV, *"...the changing skin and insides..."* that result from missed or irregular treatment, leading to poor treatment response by the patient.

- **Drink (Alcohol or beer)** and TRADITIONAL MEDICINES not to be taken together or mixed with the anti-HIV drugs

- **Diseases** such as tuberculosis, diabetes, epilepsy, hypertension and others must be discussed in relation to anti-HIV drugs as the TREATMENT being taken for these other conditions might affect the power of the anti-HIV drugs to work properly in the body.

- **Dual or double infections** with TUBERCULOSIS (TB) and how to treat the patient who has both TB and HIV infection or HIV infection followed by TB.

- **"Dangerous"** or *"...POISONOUS"* drugs that some people were saying these drugs were. These drugs are SAFE when taken as prescribed. They are NOT poisons. These medicines like all other drugs may have some side-effects that can be controlled.

- **Death** could be AVOIDED with these drugs, so long as treatment is started at the right time and the clients adhere to the treatment, no matter how inconveniencing. The Athlone Hospital staff witnessed the *"Lazarus effect"* in many patients. People who were near to death, recovered, *"...rose from the dead"* and went back to their normal lives. Many people living with HIV infection or AIDS volunteered to help the communities in local HIV infection and AIDS programmes as teachers, AIDucators, positive speakers, counsellors and buddies.

Cumberland Hotel AIDucation Report

From September 2001 to December 2001, Athlone hospital ran six "five-day long" Antiretroviral Therapy Sensitisation Workshops for five organisations that came to Lobatse, from the four initial districts that were to start providing these drugs in February 2002. Two hundred *"hands on"* participants came from:

- Botswana Network of People living with HIV infection and AIDS (BONEPWA) -35 participants in the first group

- Botswana Network of People living with HIV infection and AIDS (BONEPWA) – 25 participants in the second group

163

- Botswana Christian AIDS Intervention Programme (BOCAIP) – 30 participants in the third group
- Total Community Mobilisation (TCM) – 35 participants in the fourth group
- Healthcare workers (Nurses, doctors, pharmacists, lab technicians, nutritionists and social workers) – 35 participants in the fifth group
- Healthcare workers (Nurses, doctors, pharmacists, laboratory technicians, nutritionists, VCT counsellors and social workers) - 40 participants in the sixth group.

Athlone Hospital failed to AIDucate the teachers from the Ministry of Education as they were busy marking the final school term examination papers and therefore could not come for the social intercourse. Teachers, like social workers, are very important team players in AIDucation and raising awareness in the community.

It was five days of comprehensive AIDucation delivered with pictures and videos. It was AIDucation at its best. It was five days of the still pictures and moving pictures talking to all the groups of participants. It was five days of AIDucation, AIDucation and more AIDucation. It was five days of participants marvelling at the "National Athlone Hospital AIDS Programme." The feed back from the evaluation forms that were given in by the participants on the fifth day, last day, said it all, *"Athlone Hospital is number one!"*

Participants went back to their facilities or organisations depressed on realising how much of HIV infection and AIDS information they did not have or know. The gravity of Botswana's HIV infection and AIDS epidemics dawned on many, who had thought, that public health programmes like Athlone Hospital's were *"...making too much noise over nothing!"*

The recommendations by ALL THE GROUPS that came to Cumberland Hotel pointed in one direction, *"...Athlone Hospital's Pictures in AIDucation programme to be made national as a matter of urgency."*

In 2001, the Botswana government and its international partners began to replicate the Athlone *"...best practice"* Health Resource Centre nation wide into its twenty four health districts. In some districts, the health resource centres became the antiretroviral therapy (ARV) clinics.

Athlone Health Resource Centre would lead and others would follow.

Cumberland AIDucation workshop objectives
- To involve the various partners in the planning, implementation, monitoring and evaluation of the antiretroviral therapy drugs programme

- To utilise the already established structures and systems in the community in provision of the antiretroviral therapy drugs

- To strengthen and integrate the various organisations in comprehensive HIV infection and AIDS prevention, care and support activities

- To share information on two of the *"...best practices in Botswana,"* the Athlone AIDS Awareness Programme and the Athlone Health Resource Centre

- To identify our roles in HIV infection and AIDS prevention, care and support activities, as individuals and as members of various groups in the community.

Cumberland AIDucation workshop participants

The workshop participants were from Botswana Network of People living with HIV infection and AIDS, Botswana Christian Intervention Programme, Total Community Mobilisation and Voluntary Counselling and Testing centres. The last two groups were of healthcare workers from the four selected hospital sites of Gaborone, Serowe, Francistown and Maun. These were the four sites that would start providing antiretroviral therapy in Botswana.

Community mobilisation and sensitisation is very important before the introduction of antiretroviral drugs in any community. An AIDucated community is the secret to the success of the antiretroviral therapy programme in the village.

Cumberland AIDucation facilitators

- Athlone AIDS Awareness Project Team comprised of three nurses, three social workers and one medical doctor

- District Health Team (DHT), Lobatse Town Council, social worker, who was in charge of the Home Based Care Programme

- DHT, Lobatse Town Council, social worker, who was in charge of the Orphans and vulnerable children's Care Programme

- Guest speakers from the nutrition, laboratory and pharmacy departments in the local area, and NOT from headquarters. Aiming for local ownership.

Cumberland AIDucation presentations

The presentations fell under five general headings:

1. Basic facts on HIV infection and AIDS
2. Clinical manifestations of HIV infection and AIDS

3. Counselling, care and support

4. Antiretroviral therapy

5. Community mobilisation.

The Cumberland AIDucation course content

The AIDucation course was kept very simple and basic with room for a lot of dialogue, talking. The idea was to engage all the participants into discussions about the management of HIV infections and AIDS related matters at their sites or work stations. The course consisted:

Day 1: Social intercourse

- Introductions. House-keeping. Ground-rules. Objectives
- Fears, hopes and expectations
- Shared experiences in HIV infection and AIDS prevention, care and support activities
- Overview of global HIV infection and AIDS numbers
- **Pictures in AIDucation:** Sexually transmitted infections
- *VIDEO: Taking it home. Socio-economic impact. Stigmatisation. Arrogance of High Achievers (Zambia)*
- **Pictures in AIDucation:** Basic HIV facts, transmission and prevention.

Day 2: Clinical manifestations and antiretroviral therapy

- Recap of previous day's activities
- **Pictures in AIDucation:** Manifestations of HIV infection and AIDS in adults and children
- *VIDEO: No Need To Blame (Zimbabwe)*
- Launch of antiretroviral therapy in Botswana
- Basic facts on antiretroviral therapy
- Draft – Botswana antiretroviral therapy guidelines
- Challenges and how to improve adherence to treatment
- *VIDEO: Remember Mpho (Botswana).*

DAY 3: Counselling and emotional support

- Recap of previous day's activities
- Counselling

- **Pictures in AIDucation:** HIV infection and AIDS prevention and counselling
- Voluntary Counselling and Testing (VCT) Services
- *VIDEO: HIV infection and AIDS Counselling – The TASO Experience (Uganda)*
- Role of the Social Worker in a world of HIV infection and AIDS
- *VIDEO: Challenges in Counselling (Zambia)*
- Testimony of person living with HIV infection or AIDS.

Day 4: Support and Care Programmes
- Recap of previous day's activities
- Community Home-based Care Programme
- TB prevention and treatment
- Prevention of Mother To Child Transmission of HIV
- Nutrition in HIV infection and AIDS
- *VIDEO: Bobirwa Home-based Care Programme (Botswana)*
- Pastoral Care – *"The Good Samaritan"*
- *VIDEO: The Orphans' Generation (Uganda).*

Day 5: Community mobilisation
- Recap of previous day's activities
- Culture, sex and religion
- Community mobilisation. The Dakar Declaration
- Visit Athlone Hospital Health Resource Centre
- Recommendations and the way forward
- Evaluation. END.

LESSONS LEARNT FROM THE 2001 CUMBERLAND, BOTSWANA, ART SENSITISATION AIDUCATION WORKSHOPS
- Nothing is impossible where there is the will and the heart, despite the limited resources
- The Athlone AIDS Awareness Programme can be duplicated locally and internationally

- "Pictures in AIDucation" can be used as a teaching style, easily, in Africa and Europe as proven by the African AIDucation experience and the European AIDucation experience of Dr Edwin Mapara. Whoever thought that these slides in Cumberland Hotel, Botswana would one day be used to AIDucate folks in;
    - The United Kingdom - Birmingham, Cambridge, Leicester, London, Norwich, Oxford, and Reading
    - Cambridge University, National Institute of African Studies, Thames Valley University and University of London.
- The Athlone Health Resource Centre (AHRC) Voluntary Counselling and Testing Centre (VCT) can be duplicated locally and internationally
    - The AHRC has been replicated at Community Health Action Trust (CHAT), Willesden, London where the modified version is called Community Resource Centre
    - In an August 2007 London publication sponsored by the Medical Research Council (MRC) and the University College London (UCL), the "AHRC Model (Africa)" or rather "CHAT Model (Europe)" has been documented as "Option 2" in terms of encouraging local community based organisations to set up VCTs. There are two researched options in the report. Option 1 is for the General Practioners' (GP) Clinics or Surgeries. Option 2 ("Athlone Hospital") is for the community based organisations.
- The "Developing Countries (Third world)" can AIDucate the "Developed Countries (First world)". Programme managers should take note of the south teaching the north especially in HIV infection and AIDS related matters.

AIDUCATION

Universal precautions, including washing of hands and safe disposal of waste must be promoted in the health facilities and in home care programmes as we nurse and look after our infected loved ones. VCT stands for Voluntary Counselling and Testing. Simply walk to the nearest VCT and request for an HIV test. In some cases, the rapid finger prick test can show you your results within 20 minutes. A VCT visit can be the beginning of a new chapter in your sexual life.

12. FEARS, HOPES AND EXPECTATIONS

> *"It is the calm and silent water that drowns a man."*

African saying

Social intercourse on first day

The eight weeks of AIDucation workshops was very successful and fruitful. Athlone Hospital always began the first day with *"Fears, hopes and expectations."* This presentation always gave direction of the following days proceedings. Each group of participants talked about their fears. When the fears were exhausted, we moved on to talk about hopes and expectations. These discussions helped us to gauge the level of AIDucation knowledge of the participants.

1. Fears by Botswana Network of People living with HIV infection and AIDS (BONEPWA)

- *"No public education on the drugs"*
- *"Taking the drugs for life"*
- *"What will happen if we stop taking the drugs?"*
- *"How to tell my children living with HIV their status and my status"*
- *"Confusion among healthcare workers. No knowledge on antiretroviral therapy (ART)"*
- *"Lack of involvement of people living with HIV infection"*
- *"Silence on HIV infection and AIDS"*
- *"No networking"*
- *"Orphans will suffer"*
- *"Silence of the 300, 000 people living with HIV infection and AIDS"*
- *"Lack of successful local AIDS programmes to learn from"*
- *"Men not visible, not educated on HIV infection and AIDS, yet control sexual matters"*
- *"Donors and investors leaving the country"*
- *"ART programmes run by foreigners. Where are the locals? What about sustainability when the foreigners go away?"*
- *"Not enough food baskets"*
- *"Alcohol intake with ART"*
- *"Not responding to ART"*
- *"Stigmatisation and no confidentiality"*

169

- *"Traditional treatment mixed with ART"*
- *"Lack of counselling services"*
- *"Rural areas left out yet most of the patients will be nursed in the rural areas, the cattle-posts"*
- *"Youth not practising safer sex"*
- *"Lack of support in the villages"*
- *"No alternative treatment"*
- *"No confidence in healthcare workers"*
- *"Sex education in schools is lacking and more young people will become infected"*
- *"Gossip and revealing of secrets of house-holds by the young volunteers in home-based care"*
- *"More workshops for the educated and non-infected, yet there are more people living with HIV infection and AIDS who are not educated, poor and not working like us"*
- *"No behaviour change"*
- *"Treatment out of desperation and fear"*
- *"People will forget that prevention is better than cure"*
- *"Sharing treatment in family where there is more than one client with HIV infection. I know of such a family."*
- *"Nothing for us without us"*
- *"Lack of comprehensive information and education in the communities"*
- *"Prevention activities will be side-lined as people become excited with treatment"*
- *"Poor drug compliance because of side-effects, which are not explained properly"*
- *"People living with HIV infection and AIDS left out in ART care, yet we understand the disease better as we live with the virus every day"*
- *"Wrong people running the programme that are not compassionate and not committed."*

2. Fears by Botswana Christian AIDS Intervention Programme (BOCAIP)

- *"Death, death and more deaths"*
- *"Poor adherence to ART"*
- *"No change in behaviour as cure has been found"*
- *"Increased number of orphans and street children"*
- *"The churches not very involved, yet we are burying many of our congregation members"*
- *"Silence of the church and the ministers. Silence of the congregations."*

- *"Ignorance of AIDS and ART in the church"*
- *"Denial and judgemental attitude"*
- *"Loss of intellectuals and skilled manpower"*
- *"Crippled economy. Most of the budget will go to AIDS Programmes."*
- *"Increased deaths by carers as they become infected due to lack of knowledge"*
- *"Increased risk taking by well clients"*
- *"The hypocrisy of some churches"*
- *"Fear to take clients home from hospitals. I have been in such a situation before"*
- *"For how long will this AIDS go on?"*
- *"A lot of outside AIDS consultants in the name of AIDS while locals are left out"*
- *"Jobs created for foreigners while locals left out"*
- *"Not enough information on treatment with the public"*
- *"Workshops are only in towns and cities. Coming to Lobatse is a change for a national workshop. Usually such workshops are held in Gaborone."*
- *"Traditional doctors will stop ART so as to stop side effects on people living with AIDS"*
- *"Media involvement is minimal"*
- *"Churches and spiritual healers that claim to heal AIDS"*
- *"Delayed counselling and testing of clients"*
- *"Erratic ART doses as clients identify drugs causing bad side-effects and only choose to drink those tablets with no side-effects, like they do for hypertension"*
- *"Lack of public-private partnerships"*
- *"Lack of local word for therapy. Confusion. Cure and treatment have the same Setswana word. Wrong interpretation of being treated but not cured!"*
- *"Fear of minimal involvement of non-government organisations (NGO) as Ministry of Health tries to implement the ART Programme by itself as usual. These workshops are a surprise, it has never happened before! We are usually informed in hurried meetings as stake-holders."*
- *"Starting the ART programme before all people in AIDS activities are educated, especially the traditional doctors. The traditional doctors must also come here for sensitisation and education"*
- *"Botswana being stigmatised as "Number one" in the world. Batswana students studying abroad are being stigmatised"*

- *"Resignation of health-care workers for "greener pastures" and so the programmes are left with no implementers"*
- *"Not enough counselling facilities in both the urban and rural areas"*
- *"Raising the hopes of the people, but fail to deliver ART"*
- *"I just fear. As people talk of their fears, I become depressed and more depressed. Botswana has a bleak future. People are still to die in thousands. Our young people will be wiped out. Lord have mercy on us!"*
- *"Amen, amen and amen!"*

3. Fears by the healthcare workers

- *"ART seen as a cure"*
- *"Mystery and secrecy around the ART Project, seems to be for a few chosen healthcare workers"*
- *"Nutrition not addressed in relation to ART"*
- *"Resistant strains of HIV will develop"*
- *"Sharing treatment in family"*
- *"PMTCT confusion and now more confusion with ART"*
- *"No security. Drugs will be stolen"*
- *"Drug interactions with traditional medicines"*
- *"Lack of information amongst healthcare workers about what is happening"*
- *"Rushed programme. We do not know what is happening!"*
- *"Healthcare workers talking about compliance instead of adherence with ART"*
- *"Lack of commitment by service providers"*
- *"Migration of population to sites where ART is being given"*
- *"Abuse by healthcare workers who are HIV positive"*
- *"Prevention programmes and other public health programmes losing out"*
- *"Lack of infrastructure to put ART in place"*
- *"No laboratory equipment"*
- *"Cultural beliefs that spread HIV transmission not being addressed"*
- *"Centralised programme. We need to decentralise"*
- *"No education on adherence to public"*
- *"Selling of drugs by patients so as to buy basic commodities such as food"*

- *"Few and far away voluntary counselling and testing centres"*
- *"No patient tracking and monitoring systems in place"*
- *"Illegal pharmacists and quacks trading in ART"*
- *"The criteria for choosing patients for ART"*
- *"There are more questions than answers for ART"*
- *"Stress on ART and silence on prevention strategies. Healthcare workers also making same mistake"*
- *"Psychological impact on people who do not qualify for ART"*
- *"Lack of involvement of people living with HIV infection and AIDS who can be good adherence counsellors and role models"*
- *"Bureaucracy and red tape"*
- *"Marginalisation of traditional doctors and spiritual healers who can be good adherence counsellors"*
- *"Stigma and failure to address stigma"*
- *"Poverty and socio-economic status of clients"*
- *"No net-working with other government bodies and NGOs"*
- *"Private doctors left out, yet they started providing ART before government"*
- *"Population increase as pregnancy will be passport to ART for desperate would be mothers"*
- *"No aggressive media involvement"*
- *"Sustainability of ART Project. How long will the government sustain the bill when the other partners go away?"*
- *"Newspapers write more on football than on AIDS which is serious"*
- *"Lack of laboratory personal involvement. It is my first time today to attend an AIDS workshop in my five years of working for government"*
- *"Lack of transport to ferry clients to treatment centres"*
- *"Shortage of social workers, lab technicians, nurses, pharmacists, pharmacy technicians, counsellors, medical doctors, nutritionists, dieticians and physiotherapists"*
- *"Conflict (Professional versus personal) by healthcare workers on whether to treat or not to treat non-citizens as these drugs are for citizens. What do we do with the Maparas?"*
- *"Healthcare workers playing God. Choose who lives and who dies"*
- *"ART drugs will be found on the black market"*
- *"No commitment by stake – holders"*

173

- *"Cross border trade in ART"*
- *"Suspicions about ART drugs"*
- *"Conspiracy theories about ART"*
- *"Starting at 4 sites instead of at least 12 sites. There will be a lot of movement to these four sites by patients."*

HOPES AND EXPECTATIONS

Combined comments from all the year 2001 AIDucation participants

- *"Not just another workshop"*
- *"Flexibility of ART"*
- *"Cure to be found"*
- *"Changing of attitudes towards AIDS epidemic"*
- *"Recruit more healthcare workers"*
- *"Normalise AIDS and reduce stigmatisation"*
- *"Health education and workshops in rural areas"*
- *"Mainstream AIDS activities"*
- *"For the churches to learn the facts"*
- *"The schools to seriously address AIDS and not just as biology lesson"*
- *"Your pictures of 1997 tour in the hospitals to be given to all the hospitals, schools and churches, so that we all speak the same language on AIDS"*
- *"Network should be practical and not theoretical"*
- *"Appropriate local messages for AIDS awareness"*
- *"Behaviour change and adherence to ART to be emphasised"*
- *"Orphans will be looked after as our children"*
- *"Cultural practices that spread AIDS to be re-visited. We must talk about these bad practices."*
- *"The Catholic Church to promote condom use so as to save lives. Many churches will answer for the blood and souls lost to AIDS. The day of judgement is coming. Many church leaders will be held accountable!"*
- *"Strict audit. Changes to be made if need be whenever necessary. Not to wait for one year"*
- *"People will turn to God in prayers, as '...my people perish due to lack of knowledge...' says the Bible"*
- *"Need for clarity of roles by all in distribution of these AIDS drugs"*

- *"Kasane will have similar workshops. There is a disaster in Kasane!"*

- *"Government to support community initiatives that have done very well such as Bobirwa, Gabane, Ramotswa and Lobatse"*

- *"Cut down on red tape, bureaucracy, when asking for funds for HIV infection and AIDS activities"*

- *"Athlone Hospital AIDucation programme to be shown on Botswana TV"*

- *"Your hospital (Athlone Hospital) to help the other hospitals to get money from Ministry of Health to run AIDS programmes like you do"*

- *"Government officers to be surcharged for not spending AIDS' money that is for community programmes"*

- *"Health resource centres will be built in other hospitals and churches"*

- *"Make AIDucation a degree programme at University of Botswana (UB) in the Social Sciences. There is no AIDS course at UB. In South Africa, UNISA (University of South Africa) has an AIDS Course."*

- *"Not only at UB. Make AIDucation a diploma course in all international universities. With globalisation, we are still to die in the millions, because people do not know about AIDS like you do."*

- *"More belief and confidence in ourselves and less in foreign consultants. Look at Athlone AIDS Programme! At such times I am proud to be a Motswana."*

- *"Politicians and traditional leaders must attend these AIDucation sessions here. Some of the politicians give contradicting messages. One politician said that a fat person cannot have AIDS."*

AIDUCATION

Window period can be anything between 4 weeks to 12 weeks or even more. What is the *"window period"* in a world of HIV infection and AIDS? Is the *"window period"* the same for HIV type 1 and HIV type 2?

X-rays have a role to play in the diagnosis of tuberculosis (TB) and HIV infection. Leave it to your doctor or nurse who will do what is expected to make a diagnosis of TB and HIV infection in the patient. TB is related to HIV infection and AIDS. HIV infection and AIDS are related to TB.

13. Shared experiences in AIDS activities

Unless you call out, who will open the door?"

African saying

1. Centres of *"best practice"* activities in Botswana

All the health facilities and other institutions like the churches shared their experiences at their sites of operation. The most notable ones were the Voluntary Counselling and Testing Centre in Maun, Bamalete Lutheran Hospital in Ramotswa, the Infectious Diseases Clinic at Princess Marina Hospital in Gaborone and the Athlone Hospital Health Resource Centre in Lobatse.

The Voluntary Counselling and Testing Centre in Maun

Maun voluntary counselling and testing centre stood out in its local initiatives to encourage people to know their status, by going for an HIV test. The centre has a strong working relationship and network with Botswana Christian AIDS Intervention Programme (BOCAIP). The participants from Maun spoke very highly about the centre and its partnership with the faith communities and the solid referral system which was working very well. The Maun VCT and the faith communities were *"...hand in glove"* said one Maun participant.

The Bamalete Lutheran Hospital in Ramotswa

Bamalete Lutheran Hospital in Ramotswa received a round of applause for its hospice, the Day Care Centre, the AIDS Programme and for its committee that works with about twenty traditional doctors, faith healers and spiritual healers. In fact Bamalete Lutheran Hospital even had a referral system with the traditional healers, faith healers and spiritual healers. In most health facilities, traditional doctors are part of the problem whereas in Ramotswa, traditional doctors were part of the solution.

The Infectious Disease Clinic in Princess Marina Hospital

The Princess Marina Hospital clinic was discussed at length. The Harvard research arm and the ART arm were not well defined. The staffing and logistics of the infectious disease clinic left many participants feeling that Princess Marina Hospital was far from ready and that there was an element of uncertainty. This was further compounded by the fact that nurses did not do counselling. Counselling is the domain of social workers who are grossly understaffed.

The Athlone Health Resource Centre Team was congratulated on its *"AIDS at the workplace"* programme which was now *"...a house-hold name"* in Botswana. The programme had been in existence for almost eleven years and had conducted training sessions for almost all government ministries and departments. For a district hospital, it was observed that Athlone Hospital had done better than many hospitals, including surpassing some referral hospitals in AIDucation. Athlone Hospital's dedication, commitment and vision were mentioned by every group that came for the AIDucation workshops in Lobatse. In terms of Pictures in AIDucation, Athlone Hospital was in *"...a league of its own"* said one of the senior citizens. Athlone Hospital was second to none in the districts in terms of the AIDS Awareness programme.

Athlone Hospital had three visiting Norwegian student nurses during the period of the AIDucation sensitisation workshops at Cumberland in 2001. They took part in the workshops and were actively involved. They expressed shock at the HIV infection and AIDS numbers in Botswana. The student nurses came from a country with a population of 4.6 million people and had about 800 cases of HIV infection or AIDS in Norway. They saw their first AIDS patients here in Botswana. The students said that they were *"...recovering from the shock of seeing so many suffering patients with AIDS in Athlone Hospital wards."* The students encouraged the participants to go an extra mile for the country of Botswana. *"You must be positive, focussed and have hope for a better future"* was their message to the participants. The students also observed that there were genuine efforts by the community to address the AIDS epidemic, *"...but they are not co-ordinated very well."*

For the records, all the workers at Athlone Hospital, that is all the nurses, paramedics, industrial class and doctors had undergone fifteen full days of AIDucation courses over the years. Their first three days basic AIDucation course was in 1994 and their last five days AIDucation course was in 2001. In fact it was no surprise when Athlone Hospital's senior social worker was appointed as the first Director of the Botswana and United States of America (BOTUSA) national Voluntary Counselling and Testing Programme in 1999, after the birth of the Athlone Health Resource Centre. He played a major role in setting up the centre in Lobatse.

Athlone Hospital in Lobatse had made its mark in the history of Botswana's HIV infection and AIDS control programmes. The success of the Athlone AIDS Awareness Programme was not due to one person, it was due to many persons. It was not due to an individual's work, it was due to team-work. It was not due to competition, it was due to cooperation. It was not due to rivalry, it was due to togetherness. The recorded success was due to one united front as we fought one common enemy called HIV infection that can lead to AIDS.

CONCLUSION

African saying

A tearful farewell

I think my early *"...alarmist..."* days in the 1990s were wonderfully and emotionally summarised by a senior nurse in Francistown, which is about five hundred miles away from Lobatse. It all happened when I was giving a farewell talk to the residents and hospital staff at Nyangabgwe Hospital, Francistown, in June 2001. This was after spending four days in Francistown, where I was a member of a consultative government team that was finding out if Francistown was ready to start providing its people living with HIV infection and AIDS antiretroviral therapy or anti-HIV drugs to improve their quality of life.

The senior nurse, in one of the meeting rooms, at about 6.00pm, on the last day, almost made us all cry. I had to hold back tears and tactfully use the opportunity to encourage the teams to be hopeful and not to despair. She said, *"Ngaka (Doctor), it breaks my heart to look at you standing there."* She paused, inhaled deeply and continued, *"In the early 1990s we used to hear a lot of 'modumo'- noise - coming from Lobatse. It was all caused by you. We asked the matron of Athlone Hospital at that time about what was happening in Lobatse.*

The matron responded by saying that "...The Ministry of Health has employed a small Zambian doctor who spends all his time talking about AIDS, AIDS and AIDS. He says that Botswana has a pending disaster...he says that the government is not doing much to stop the spread of AIDS...he says that one day Botswana will lead the world in terms of AIDS patients, surpassing countries like Uganda and Zambia...he says we shall be burying people from Monday to Monday...he says there will be thousands of orphans and street children...he says that no one will not know of a friend, relative or work colleague who will have died of AIDS...He says foreign doctors will come and take over the running of the AIDS Programmes. This small doctor even says that Athlone Hospital's AIDS Awareness Programme will play a major role in Botswana's future AIDS Programmes...Can you imagine!"

The senior nurse went on and on, with the other members of staff nodding their heads in agreement, as she recalled events that had passed, not in the distant past. As she spoke she was overcome by emotions and tears started rolling down her face, but still speaking with a steady earnest voice. It was infectious. Other nurses started sobbing and sniffing to, as tears rolled down those round

African cheeks. Hand movements were many as the nurses dried their eyes with tissues and handkerchiefs, trying to keep a brave face.

The senior nurse concluded by saying, *"Ngaka all those things that you said in the early days of the epidemic have happened. We never knew that it was going to be this bad! How many of us have not buried a relative, friend or work colleague? How many of us have not been affected by AIDS? How many of us do not know of orphans or look after orphans? How many of us have not been touched by this strange disease? How many of us do not pray every night for a better tomorrow? You spoke like a prophet! Now here you are just about to leave us for London, when we need you most!"*

Her last sentence almost melted me and I could feel the tears swelling up in my eyes, but I quickly checked myself before I was overcome by emotions. *"Boys do not cry, even big boys!"* I used this sad farewell departure to encourage all the local teams to work in overdrive and believe in themselves. It is not all doom and gloom. If a small district hospital like Athlone Hospital in Lobatse could have three documented community *"...best practices..."* HIV infection and AIDS control programmes, then other hospitals can easily do better.

On the 28th August 2002, I left the African continent for Europe. It was a mixture of emotions, sadness and joy, as I boarded the plane in Johannesburg, South Africa. At 10.00pm. I sat back in the seat with my three very excited boys, next to me, who were enjoying this adventure of flying off to Europe, to see their mother and to start a new life in London. I closed my eyes and said a farewell prayer thanking Him above for the gift of life, for my wife and friends, for the extended family, for my many friends, for the doctors and nurses, for my many clients living with HIV infection and AIDS. I thanked God for having provided our daily bread, for having sustained us and for having kept us well on the African continent. As the plane took off from the African soil, warm tears rolled down my cheeks. Good-bye Zambia, good-bye Botswana, good-bye South Africa, good-bye Mother Africa. There is hope for Africa, so long as *African communities talked sex, AIDS and pictures.*

AIDUCATION

Youth and adults should work together for a better tomorrow. The Ethiopians say, *"One spider's web cannot tie up a lion. Many spiders' webs can tie up even the strongest lion!"*

Zero or *"undetectable levels"* means you have very low levels of HIV in the blood. Despite the very low concentration or "undetectable levels" of the virus in the body, one still remains HIV positive and can still infect other people.

REFERENCES

There are some online articles or internet papers that refer to Dr Edwin Mavunika Mapara and Pictures in AIDucation or the Athlone Hospital AIDS Awareness Project, Lobatse, Botswana:

A. AIDS is in the village, the strategies are in the village
    o   http:bmj.bmjjournals.com/cgi/eletters/329/7457/67-a

B. Botswana: Shock visual tactics prove successful in AIDS education
    o   http://www.aegis.com/news/irin/2005/IR050235.html

C. Comment: SADC Report on HIV Prevention
    o   http://eforums.healthdev.org/read/messages?id=13199

D. Don't let things slide!
    o   http:www.talcuk.org/free/html/am_3/am.htm

E. Eforums comment: Pictures as Health Promotion strategy
    o   http://eforums.healthdev.org/eforums/cms/showMessage.asp?msgid=5560

F. Female condoms
    o   http://www.healthdev.org/eforums/cms/showMessage.asp?msgid=7884

G. Global AIDS: Declare war on HIV/AIDS
    o   http://www.aids.net.au/aids-global-png-aidswar.htm

H. HIV/AIDS and teachers in Africa
    o   http://eforums.healthdev.org/read/messages?id=5294

I. Initiating a blood transfusion
    o   http://bmj.bmjjournals.com/cgi/eletters/329/7461/308-a

J. Jerry Rawlings' entourage in Botswana
    o   http://forums.comminit.com/viewtopic.php?p=186241

K. Kubatana net: Pictures as a health promotion strategy
    o   http://www.kubatana.net/html/archive/health/040519health.asp?sector=health&year=...

L. ...Local Public Health issues are in the hands of the local communities
    o   http://www.healthdev.org/viewmsgid=893b6a8d-16b8-4149-afbb-bf6342e0...

M. Money spinning venture for HIV/AIDS consultants
    o   http://forums.comminit.com/viewtopic.php?p=186241

N. New SAVE strategy better than ABC
    o   http://www.ahpn.org/news/clipings/index.php?clipping_id=66

O. Opinion: Pictures as a health promotion
    o   www.safaids.org.zw/publications/SAFAIDS%20NEWS%20SEPTEMBER.pdf

P. Picturing AIDS: Using images to raise community awareness
    o   http://medicine.plosjournals.org/peent&doi=3D10.1371/journal.pmed.0010043

Q. (Questions and) Solutions are in the hands of the local communities

    o   http://www.healthdev.org/viewmsg.aspx?msgid=893b6a8d-6b8-4149-afbb-bf6342e0...

R. Ratings and comments on Pictures in AIDucation

    o   http://www.cominit.com/healthecomm/top-tens.php?showdetails=188

S. Sub-Saharan countries have nothing to lose and all to gain by HIV counselling and testing of all TB patients

    o   http://bcm.thaimalil.com/mywebboard/readmess.php3?user=noktpr&idroom=1&idforum=...

T. TB discussion with Thailand colleagues

    o   http://bcm.thaimail.com/mywebboard/readness.php3?user=noktpr&idroo=1&idforum=...

U. Universal "3x5" – A Wish or a Reality

    o   http://bmjjournals.com/cgi/eletters/328/7449/1151

V. Voluntary counselling and testing

    o   www.ahpn.org/news/clippings/index.php?clipping_id=66

W. What is and in a condom?

    o   http://bmjjournals.com/cgi/eletters/329/7459/185

X. X-rated article: Popularizing female condoms

    o   http://www.healthdev.org/eforums/cms/showMessage.asp?msgid=7884

Y. Young Fabians Society article on donor aid to developing countries

    o   http://forums.comminit.com/viewtopic.php?p=186241

Z. Zambian HIV/AIDS background

    o   http://forums.comminit.com/viewtopic.php?p=186241